Betty

From Slyne Head to Malin Head,
A Rural GP Remembers.

Ron O'Flaherty

First Published in Ireland 2003

by author Ken O'Flaherty

Cover and Illustrations by Bridget Murray

Printed by Browne Printers Letterkenny

ISBN: 0-9546312-0-X

DEDICATION

I wish to dedicate this book to my wife Eileen.

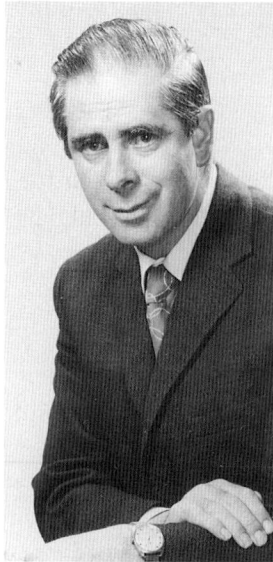

ACKNOWLEDGEMENTS

I would like to thank the following;
Typist, Agnes Keaveney and Marie Quigg, proof readers, Séan Beatty, Edward and Mary O'Kane, Helen McLaughlin and Bernadette Cannon and Serenity House, Moville for all their help. A special thanks goes to Bridget Murray for her beautiful illustrations.

A percentage of the profits will be donated to the Alzheimer's Society of Ireland and the Foyle Hospice, Derry.

Why I Wrote This Book

As I was approaching retirement in the early eighties, I began to look back over my life and recall memories that had almost vanished during my hectic years as a single-handed general medical practitioner. I gradually began to consider writing some form of record when I would retire in 1990; eventually in the year 2000 I decided it was time to start at least a family history or at most a memoir/autobiography. In that millennium year I had written an article published in the Irish Medical Times (a weekly publication) and another article written for UCD Connections (a worldwide annual magazine for college alumni). The publication of these two articles was the catalyst that persuaded me to take the plunge to write a full memoir/autobiography of my life and experiences as I saw them from the early thirties to the year 2002.

All of this time taking in a large part of the twentieth century, the threat of World War 2 in the early thirties to the actual war from 1939 to 1945. In the forties and fifties, the epidemics of poliomyelitis and tuberculosis, the rapid speeding up of rural electrification, the advances in radio and television leading on to computers where the technology is endless. From the sixties and seventies, huge advances in medicine, organ transplants and an avalanche of new therapeutic drugs. On the downside there are the alcoholic and drug cultures which are causing intolerable pressure on hospitals and other resources.

On leaving Ballyconneely National School, I went to a secondary boarding school in Dublin where I witnessed the North Strand bombing. Despite all the discomforts of wartime Dublin, I enjoyed my time there. On the day I got my Leaving Cert results was the day after the bombs were dropped on Hiroshima and Nagasaki.

Having three uncles, two granduncles and six first cousins all doctors, I studied medicine in UCD. Half way through the course I got tuberculosis but, thanks to a very early diagnosis, I recovered rapidly. During my college years I enjoyed Dublin student life and also enjoyed the long summer holidays in Ballyconneely and assisting my brother and workmen saving turf on the bog and hay in the meadows. All of the family took stints in the bar although none of us liked the drinks culture.

Having graduated in 1952, finished hospital and engaged to Eileen, one day, out of the blue, I was offered a private medical practice with rented accommodation in Moville, Co Donegal, literally on the shores of Lough Foyle in the Inishowen Peninsula. Eileen and myself had planned to emigrate to England for a while but the moment we got this offer we could not refuse it. I was confident that I had gained very practical experience in the four hospitals where I had trained in that era. In addition Eileen and myself loved the sea and countryside so we would have no problem in putting down roots in Inishowen.

Contents

Prologue

I was born in Seamount Nursing Home in Salthill, Galway on 27th October 1926. I am determined to pass on this information in the opening statement in this work because I have always held the conviction that keeping one's age a secret is a most futile exercise. I was the second of three children; my brother Bernard was three years older and my sister Carmel, yet-to-come, would be eight and a half years younger.

My father Tom O'Flaherty inherited a pub and grocery business and an attached farm in Ballyconneely five and a half miles west of Clifden, Co Galway. My grandfather Tom O'Flaherty, had married into an O'Malley family who I presume owned the business and farm. My mother Imelda Lee, was born into a similar background of a pub, grocery and farming business in Clifden.

In the twenties and thirties while Ireland was recovering from The War of Independence and the Civil War that followed, business and professional people like the legal, medical, teaching engineering and other professions were relatively secure so I was fortunate to have been born into a stratum of society in which there was a reasonable standard of living and almost a guarantee of a second and third-level education providing I had the wit to grasp the opportunities which were there for the taking.

My grandmother on my father's side was an O'Malley. Some of that family were in the legal profession; one of them, William O'Malley, was a Barrister and an M.P. for Connemara and as far as I could ascertain was a supporter of Parnell and Redmond. There were six children in the O'Flaherty family, Tom my father; Kathleen who trained as a nurse in the Mater Hospital in Dublin. She served in the 1914 – 1918 war in the RAMC. After the war she emigrated to Los Angeles and later moved on to Hawaii where she worked for many years in a hospital attached to a pineapple plantation. She died in Waikiki around 1958; Agnes married a businessman in Dingle Co Kerry; Alice married the Chief Engineer of the Marconi Telegraphy Station situated near a bog in Derrygimla between Clifden and Ballyconneely; Nellie died from T.B. in her youth; Michael the youngest became a Doctor and emigrated to England and Scotland but lost touch with the family.

There were eight children in my mother's family, four girls and four boys. May, the eldest, married Dr. Joe Casey who was the dispensary doctor in Clifden; Delia married Patrick O'Malley from Cleggan; Rita studied medicine for a while but gave it up to marry a doctor, Paddy Muldoon who became a dispensary doctor in Mohill, Co Leitrim. They had four children, the youngest Paddy was not yet born when his father was shot dead during the Civil War. The four boys in the Lee family were James who took over the business; Ambrose who became a solicitor and died at a young age in 1934; Michael studied medicine and became a Dispensary Doctor in Newport, Co Mayo; Alfred also studied medicine and he emigrated to England.

Marconi and Alcock and Brown

The Marconi Station already mentioned brought a certain amount of prosperity to the Clifden and Ballyconneely area.

When Gugliema Marconi, the Italian Pioneer of wireless telegraphy, decided to search for a site to build a transmission station somewhere along the Atlantic coast of Ireland (so that it would be possible to send messages without cables across the Atlantic) he eventually decided on Derrygimla three miles outside Clifden on the Ballyconneely road. The site chosen was on the edge of a widespread peat bog land ironically spreading towards the Roundstone bog, which in recent times has been seriously considered as a site for a small airport.

In 1905 construction commenced and this must have been a great boost for the economy of the Clifden and Ballyconneely areas. Very large buildings were required for the running of the proposed station when completed and several dwelling houses for the resident staff of engineers and technicians.

My Aunt Alice and husband lived there for some time in the Chief Engineer's bungalow, which was built, with a bright red roof. As expected the area was very cold and exposed to the winds blowing in from the Atlantic so they called it 'Cold Blow'. I have vivid memories of the many times the couple mentioned 'Cold Blow' whenever they visited Ballyconneely in the thirties.

Up to this time 'Cold Blow' was still there and its bright red roof was clearly visible from the main road between Ballinaboy and Errislanin.

A small narrow gauge railway was built from the main road to the station complex for transporting building materials and equipment including two large masts for transmission.

As large quantities of fuel were required for powering many generators it was decided to use turf (peat) in preference to coal as the site was beside a vast bog so for this reason a large force of men was employed to cut and save the turf during the spring and summer months. Seventy or more men were employed every year and this was a huge economic boost for the area. The station was officially opened in 1907 and the first commercial wireless messages were transmitted across the Atlantic to Cape Breton in Canada.

By now Derrygimla had officially gone into the history books, and the microchip was on its way but there was another first about to occur in Derrygimla. Twelve years later on Sunday morning 15th June 1919 a small aeroplane came flying in over the Atlantic and passing near Slyne Head flew northwards near the coastline of Errismore and then flying in over Clifden.

The two airmen on board observed the two high masts at Marconi's station and assumed that the surrounding area would be a suitable landing place. They came in to land but the wheels of the aeroplane sank into the soft bog causing the nose of the plane also to go into the soft surface thus ended the momentous and historic first flight to cross the Atlantic from the West to East. Derrygimla was in the history books for the second time. The two brave airmen, John Arthur Alcock and Whitten Brown, escaped injury and were able to enjoy a hearty Irish breakfast with my Aunt Alice and her husband in 'Cold Blow' on that historic Sunday morning.

My father clearly remembered the loud sound of the plane as it passed Slyne Head to Errismore that morning. One of my great regrets is that I had an original photograph of the crashed plane for many years but unfortunately it is now lost. It is a well-known fact that large parts of the plane were taken away for souvenirs before the authorities whisked it away to London to be repaired before moving it to an aviation museum.

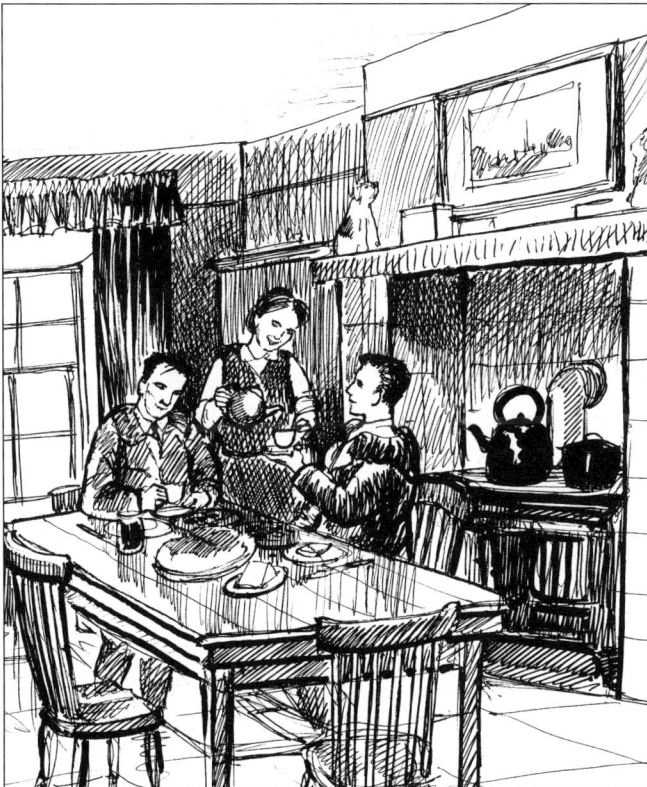

From Slyne Head to Malin Head, A Rural GP Remembers.

Civil War

During the height of the Civil War two men called to our house in Ballyconneely. My parents were away at that time so they asked or probably demanded my grandfather to give them my father's car, a model T Ford. In the times that were in it he was in no position to refuse. Apparently the two men used the car to transport them to Marconi station to burn it down. They carried out their task but the station was not completely destroyed since it was never fully restored as by that time it was losing its importance as wireless telegraphy was progressing so rapidly it was becoming redundant. Incidentally my father's car was returned unharmed. Despite the fact that the station was becoming less important it was still employing people and when it finally closed it was a severe loss for the area.

When I was growing up in the thirties I heard many stories and experiences from men who had worked there. On a few occasions Bernard and myself, with other grown up young men, hunted hares on the Derrygimla Bog with some of the local men and when we reached the ruins of the station it was a sad and very lonely sight. We used to root around in the ruins and take away pocketfuls of small thick discs of glass, which had been used in the numerous electric batteries, used for the generation of electricity.

We kept them as souvenirs. 'Cold Blow' with its red roof was still standing and we wondered how much longer it would be there, certainly not for very long.

Despite the loss of the station West Connemara still had a developing Tourist Trade, which was some help as the area had always attracted the more wealthy English tourists.

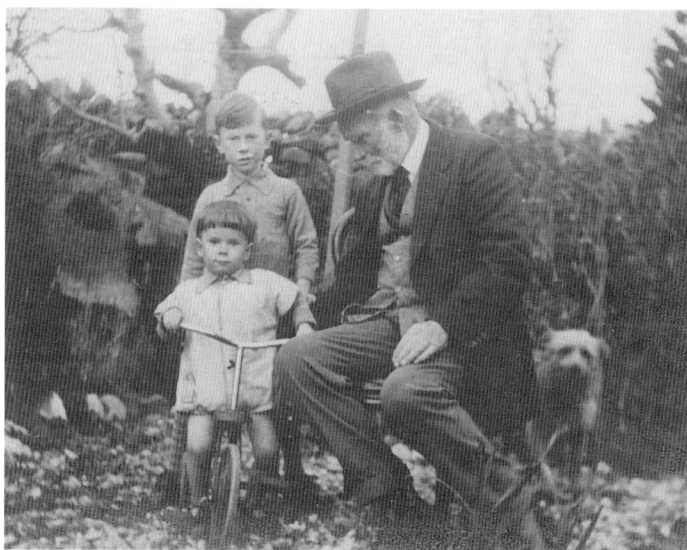

Bernard, Ken and grandfather Thomas.(1929)

The Thirties

My earliest memories go back to some time around 1931. I vaguely remember Grandfather O'Flaherty from a short time before his death in May 1931. The thirties appeared to me as being a long and exciting decade. I have a hazy memory of my mother taking me walking to Ballyconneely National School for my first day there. The school was approximately a quarter of a mile away.

Bernard could not go to school at that time due to frequent illness from an asthmatic chest and for a few years had to get tuition at home.

My first clear memory is of the Eucharistic Congress held in Dublin in 1932. In those days the Catholic faith was very strong in Ireland so for the majority of the population this would have been a time of great celebration coming at a relatively short time after the awful stress and trauma of The War of Independence and worse still the Civil War. For weeks preceding the Congress cars flew small congress flags. These were a dark blue colour with a gold coloured crest in the centre representing a Celtic cross. These little flags could be tied to the headlights of most of the cars of that era as the headlights protruded up from the mudguards, as they were called-in modern speak 'The Wings'.

Large versions of the flags were flown from windows of dwellings and from many flagpoles. Many people wore bronze coloured badges designed like a Celtic cross.

The Congress was a great success with over a million people attending the main ceremonies in the Phoenix Park, including many Catholic Church Dignitaries – sadly Ecumenism was not on the agenda at that time.

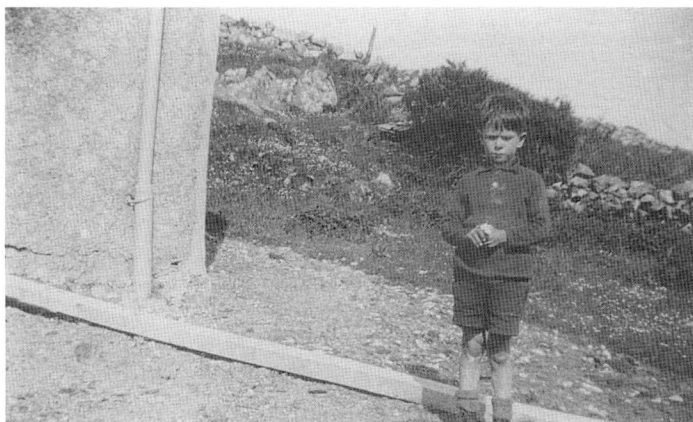

Ken.(1933)

From Slyne Head to Malin Head, A Rural GP Remembers.

Politics in the Thirties

From the time of the Treaty in 1921 the then Cumman Na Gael (later to become Fine Gael) Political party was in power led by W.T. Cosgrave. The anti-treaty party, which became Fianna Fail, led by Eamon de Valera was the main opposition party.

I have vivid memories of the 1932 election. I was then six years of age and certainly got a great insight and a great experience into what politics was all about like the church gate speeches interrupted frequently by vigorous heckling, derogatory accusations and frequent verbal re-enactments of the Civil War.

Canvassers in cars flew along the dusty roads bedecked with flags and car stickers on all the windows except the windscreen, beseeching voters to vote for the named candidate or candidates. Being born into a family that was reasonably well off, your prospects in life were better than those not so fortunate. Similarly political allegiance in those days almost invariably followed the same path as the parents. That is not the situation in modern times as people make up their own minds. Tragically we now have a situation where less and less people vote.

Election days used to be hectic and as expected it would be very busy in pubs where politics could be a flashpoint for arguments and rows. As far as I can remember while the pub in Ballyconneely would be very busy but peaceful as most people left their political views outside the door.

Fianna Fail won the 1932 election by a very small majority and was depending on support from the Labour party so in 1933 Mr. de Valera called another election, which he won by a large majority. After the 1933 election and when the new government settled into power, there was an aftermath and this political period became known as 'the time of the Blue Shirts'. This situation caused consternation among Cumman Na Gael (Fine Gael) supporters which led by General O'Duffy who founded the Blue Shirts which got its name from men supporters wearing a heavy blue shirt and women wearing a blue blouse. Cumman Na Gael alleged that the reason for founding this organisation was that Eamon de Valera after coming to power encouraged supporters to break up political meetings of the opposition party so the blue shirts were to defend Cumman Na Gael meetings. O'Duffy had a large support for a time with large meetings and parades but people became worried about the similarity of the movement to the fascist movements of Hitler, Mussolini and Franco in Europe. When the Civil War in Spain broke out O'Duffy organised a Brigade of Volunteers to go to Spain to help Franco fight against alleged communism but I am not getting involved in that one.

At that time I did not understand the whole thing but from a young man's point of view it appeared to be an exciting time and left me with vivid memories of the early thirties.

Sport

For me 1932 was also an Olympic Year and I heard from my father of the feats of the great Dr. Pat O'Callaghan who won the gold medal for throwing the hammer at the 1932 Olympics in Los Angeles. He had also won the gold medal for the hammer throwing in the Amsterdam Olympics of 1928. Irishman Bob Tisdall also won a gold medal for the high hurdles in Los Angeles. My father explained that these big games were held every four years in a different country and that the best athletes from most countries competed for the Olympic Medals.

This early introduction to sport in general and the Olympic Games in particular lit a flame in me for a love of athletics and all other sports with the exception of cricket. When the 1936 Olympics were held four years later in Berlin, Bernard and myself could read enough of the newspaper to follow the feats of the great American Jessie Owens in the sprints and long jump. Radio commentaries and news bulletins had arrived and this added to the interest. In 1936, we did not know the next Olympics were to be twelve years away in London in 1948.

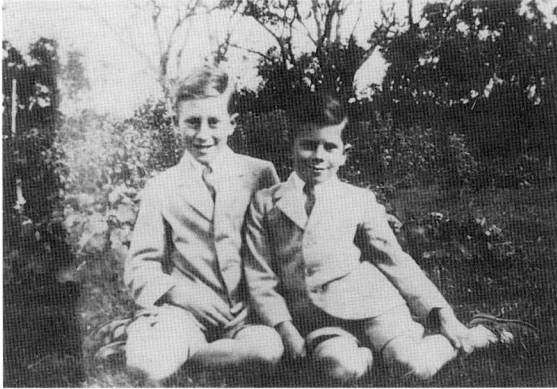

1st Communion. Ken and Bernard (1940's)

Communications in the Thirties

Regarding newspapers and their deliveries in the thirties my father got the Irish Independent daily by mail. It would have been sent by rail from Dublin to Clifden (after 1935 when the Clifden train had stopped) the mail would travel by P.O. train to Galway and then by van to Clifden where it was sorted and taken five miles to Ballyconneely Post Office by the local postman on his big P.O. bike.

This mail and paper would be delivered in Ballyconneely at 3 pm. Despite all our great advances in speed etc there has not been much change in physical postal services excepting the miracle of the E-Mail. When the postman's load was over a certain weight, a hackney car was provided to transport himself and the mail to Ballyconneely. Bernard and myself used to spread the paper on the floor to read it.

Radio

The radio or the wireless as it was then called arrived very gradually in the thirties to the few areas that had electricity supplied and then to the rural areas by means of the wet and dry batteries which necessitated recharging the wet battery very frequently, the dry battery being replaced at longer intervals. It was also necessary to have an aerial which was a wire leading into the radio. I cannot remember exactly when we got our first radio but it had to be between September 1934 and 1935. We did not have a radio when Galway defeated Dublin in the 1934. All Ireland but we did have one when Mayo beat Laois in 1935 or was it 36?

I remember the name of it was a Philco. We also got a new dog around the time and you guessed it, we called him Philco. My clearest memory is that the local priest was a radio enthusiast and dabbled in making crystal sets and had moved on to assembling real radios with valves and wires etc. One Sunday he invited a group of young people including Bernard and myself to hear a commentary of the 1934 All Ireland Final between Galway and Dublin.

This was a fantastic experience for us despite the poor sound coming through all the crackling and atmospherics. We were all dumbfounded and the fact that Galway won was the icing on the cake…

As the sound of radios improved the commentators were not keeping pace with the improvements of radios until the All Ireland Semi-final of 1938 between Galway and Monaghan when an 18-year-old lad burst on the scene and gave a brilliant commentary. This of course was Michael O'Hehir who became a famous international commentator and was famous for his commentaries on a section of the Aintree Grand National for many years. He also did the commentary on John F. Kennedy's funeral.

Ball Games

In 1938 my father brought Bernard and myself to the Connaught GAA Final between Mayo and Galway. This was a really thrilling experience for us to see the famous players in action. That final was played in Roscommon and this appeared a very long journey but a great day out. Our interests were not confined to GAA as we also followed rugby and soccer on the radio and the papers. At that stage we were playing football with our friends and played inter village matches.

During my first three to four years at school we had an elderly lady principal who would not allow us to play football in the schoolyard so the only activity was running races around the grounds. Fortunately the principle retired when I was in third class and a young male teacher called Tommy Sweeny, who was from the Ballyconneely area and had been teaching in Waterford, replaced her. Bernard and I were thrilled because he was a hero of ours from seeing him play football and running at sports meetings when he was home on holidays.

Needless to say he encouraged football and even supplied a real leather football. All leather with the rubber bladder with a nozzle which was pulled out through a small opening in the ball and then pumped usually with a bicycle pump and then bent in two and tied very tightly with a piece of string then pushed back into the ball and finally the opening which was provided with eyelets like a shoe lace and then laced up tightly. The leather part of the ball was made of numerous small sections of leather tightly sewn together from the inside so when a section ripped open from wear and tear the bladder pushed its way out through the opening, so it inevitably burst. The bladder was easily repaired like a bicycle tube but the ball required the skill of a shoemaker who turned the ball inside out and repaired the tear from the inside.

In those days our lunch was consumed under a sheltered stonewall in dry weather and inside when raining. There was no football on wet days so on dry days when football was on the agenda most of the bread was given to the seagulls who were always flying overhead to dive for their bonanza.

The teacher frequently gave us coaching on the finer arts of Gaelic as well as expertise in keeping the ball low to avoid smashing the school windows. As well as his athletic abilities he was also a good teacher and as was the norm in those days he used the slath (cane) occasionally when required. Needless to say there were no hang-ups in those days about corporal punishment. We always referred to him as 'Sweeney'. He gave Eileen and myself a barometer for a wedding present, which is still as good as new, and every time I check the weather outlook, memories come back.

Outside of school we played a lot of handball not in a proper ball alley but against a high wall that was part of a big store of the Ballyconneely premises. This wall was standing and still is along the public road so that we actually played on the road so that we had to give way to the traffic, which was not too heavy in those days. We usually played on the long summer evenings and on Sundays we used the gable end of the school. The system was that we played doubles and the winning pair of a game took on a fresh pair and so on until everybody had at least one or more games.

Hunting, Shooting and Fishing

Hunting, shooting and fishing were other activities to occupy our minds in those days. There were not everyday occurrences but usually occasional in certain seasons and days and always accompanied by adults. On St. Stephen's Day (Boxing Day) we went shooting with one or two adults who owned shotguns and walked over large areas of swampy land hoping to shoot snipe, woodcocks or wild duck or possibly an occasional hare. The men with the guns were very conscious of safety and were continuously instructing us on proper procedures in crossing drains or going over ditches or walls. Fortunately the days were at their shortest so that we survived complete exhaustion or hypothermia. Another special day was a fishing expedition and this was on Good Friday. My father was a keen fisherman in his youth when the numerous lakes and rivers in Connemara had plenty of fish. As pubs had to be closed all day on Good Friday he took Bernard and myself fishing. I felt that he looked forward to this quiet day out to get away from the inevitable pestering of small groups of people all over the country who would go to the ends of the earth to get into a pub on a closed day.
He had a big book of flies for fly-casting and we had a jar of worms. As the lakes had almost run out of fish at that time our catches would be just a few tiddlers. Please pardon the pun but I could never get hooked on lake or river fishing but I enjoyed Sea Angling. Bernard became more interested as time went on and became a member of Clifden Trout Fishing Association whose main objectives were to restock the lakes, to encourage tourists as well as encouraging local people to take up fishing. Organising fishing competitions and various social functions carried out these objectives with considerable success.

Another outdoor pastime was netting rabbits. The equipment required for this operation was a rabbit warren, at least one ferret, housed in a small square wooden box with air vents and a little flap door and a handle for carrying and last but not least a supply of string nets attached to purse strings which could be stretched out to encircle a number of rabbit burrows openings. The ideal site for a hunt was a sandy beach with sand dunes and with the purse string nets pegged into the sand around the burrows. The ferret was released and pushed into a burrow a slight distance away to hunt out the unfortunate rabbits. We the hunters then lay low behind the sand dunes and after a short time we would peep out to see if there were any struggling rabbits in the nets and when this occurred we went about our murderous task by killing the rabbit with the 'traditional rabbit punch'. This was carried out by holding up the unfortunate victim by its two hind legs and delivering a sharp quick blow with the side of the hand to the rabbit's neck to break it.

I expect this was a humane way to kill but at present I could not contemplate shooting or killing animals or birds. This rabbit hunting was carried out on the expanse of Ailbrack Beach, which is now a championship golf course.

My sister Carmel was born in May 1935, to complete the family. Having a baby in the house was a huge change and novelty for Bernard and myself due to the age difference. Bernard was twelve and I was eight and a half so life outside went on much the same but life inside was very much different.

In that year Bernard became seriously ill with pneumonia which up to that time had been a very serious illness and frequently fatal. I was horrified seeing him so ill with the doctor calling almost every day and our mother praying almost continuously. I felt extremely lonely and prayed relentlessly. Up to that time the only treatment was poulticing the chest and frequent tepid sponging to keep down the temperature and try to control the delirium. Antibiotics had not yet arrived but fortunately an anti-bacterial type of drug had recently arrived called sulphonamides. As this drug was produced and marketed by a company called May and Baker it was commonly called M. & B. and probably saved Bernard's life

To the Bog through the Fields

During the thirties electricity had not yet arrived to Ballyconneely except with vision of the local curate who in 1931- 1932 when refurbishing the Church got it wired by a local man who ran a generator on oil. This power was used only for light. The rest of the parish had to use paraffin oil lamps and candles for light and turf for heating so most households had a share of a bog on which to cut turf and save it for fuel. We had a bog about three-quarters of a mile walk through our own land. Cutting the turf was an art, which was carried out by certain men who had more strength and expertise than others. The spade used was called a shlean.

It had a sharp wing protruding up from side of the spade and coming to a point so it could be a left or right shlean to suit the operator. The natural bog would be roughly three to five feet deep consisting of wet semi-solid and pliable turf (peat). The ground on the surface covering the turf consisted of heather and various species of tough short grass extending four to six inches deep called the scraw. Before the real work began the area was marked and the surface removed with a conventional spade. In Connemara this was called 'Scrawing' the bog. The shlean man was now ready to start the real work of plunging the shlean into the soft turf and lifting the soft sods of turf on to the hard bank above.

The width and depth of the bog depended on the surrounding conditions due to rocks or excess water the width of the bog was measured by the number of sods and the depth by the length of sods each sod measured a 'spit'.

As children and youths we never attempted the expert and strenuous work of cutting the turf but we helped, as the work got lighter with the different stages of 'saving'. The freshly cut turf was first left on the ground for a short time in shallow heaps. It was then spread on the ground and at this stage, using a pitchfork or a hayfork stuck gently into each sod, carried a short distance and dropped lightly on the ground to dry in the wind and sun. It could also be moved by sticking the fingers into the wet sod. Very much depended on the vagaries of the weather when the sods would get partially dry and then the next procedure was footing the turf and that was where the children could help possibly even better than adults. The sods were by now nearly rigid so that two sods could be put upright at slights angles to support each other, then two more one on either side placed against the original pair so making the shape of a cone allowing the wind to blow freely through until depending on the weather it got completely dry. The footing was really very light for children but not so pleasant for adults and the elderly who have difficulty in stooping. There were probably different methods of saving the turf in other areas but this was the only one I had seen.

The next procedure was to get the dry turf out to the nearest bog road where it would be built into a stack along the hard ground on the side of the road and left there until it was convenient to transport it home by horse and cart. There were various ways of moving the turf to the sides of the road again depending on the weather. In very dry weather with rocky or hard ground near the bog a horse and cart could be used. A donkey and cart with rubber tyres on the wheels was very useful, as donkeys are experts at walking on soft ground. Donkeys with creels was another option, big wheel barrows another. The worst option of all after a long wet summer was humping it out in bags on human backs in squelching ground.

Working on the bog on a real summer day was a wonderful experience that will last a lifetime. The scents of the heather, the dry turf and the various bog flowers and above all the singing of the numerous skylarks continuously rising from all over the bog land always reminded me of Keats 'Ode to the Skylark' and the few lines that lingered in my memory,

> *Higher still and higher,*
> *From the earth thou springest*
> *And singing still doth soar*
> *And soaring ever singest.*

In good weather having tea breaks and lunch were real picnics. One person was delegated to boil water and make tea and hard-boiled eggs, so we peeled off the shells to enjoy them with the homemade bread and butter which always appeared to taste better on the bog. When transported home by horse and cart some of the dry turf was stored in a shed in the yard for immediate use. Most of it was built into a big stack further away.

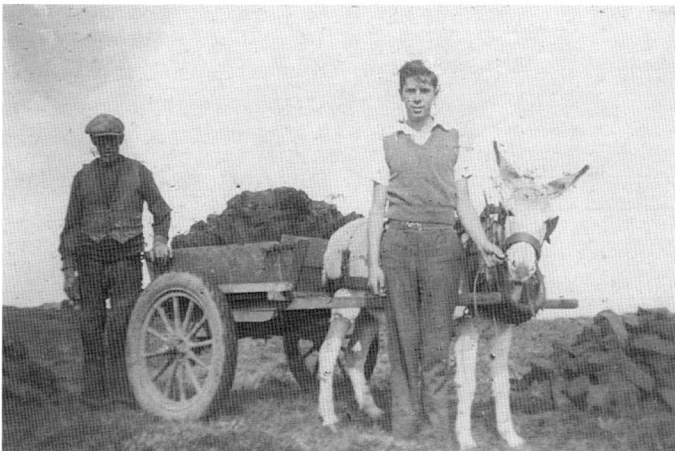

Ken and a Senior Workman in the Bog.(1942)

Modern Turf Saving

In modern times a special type of machine with massive wide tyres cuts turf. This machine cuts heather and grass as well as the raw turf and mixes up the lot and leaves the wet turf in a long roll like a string of giant sausages. When dried it is packed into large plastic fertiliser bags and left lying around the bog. Some people take a tractor load of turf home now and again and others just fill the boot of a car whenever they require it. During the winter plastic bags full of turf can be seen scattered in small heaps over the bogs.

Saving The Hay

In our younger days the hay was cut with a scythe and similar to the turf cutter there were usually expert men for that strenuous job in small wet fields where a horse drawn mowing machine could not be used. In good weather we all joined in the saving or drying process, which was carried out manually by scattering the wet green hay around with the hayforks (a long two-pronged fork).

When partially dry it was turned over in to long rolls to let the wind run through it. When drier they were made into very small cocks and eventually into much larger cocks.

This process in the very rare really good weather could be completed in four or five days while in very bad weather it could take weeks. The hay saved rapidly in good conditions would retain its green colour and fresh scent whereas that rescued in bad weather had a bleached colour and in real wet conditions it could be musty and even damp.

The large cocks of hay were left in the meadow for a few weeks before transporting to the hayshed or haystacks. To secure the cock from the wind each cock was tied down by means of a rope made from the dry hay. In Connemara this natural rope was called by its Irish name 'sugán' and there was an art in making it. One person knelt, sat or stooped at the base of the cock and gradually and gently pulled out a handful of hay and by gently teasing it out and twisting at the same time as he or she did so, it formed a short rope approximately two feet in length. This was then wrapped around the base of a hayfork handle held by another operator who rotated the fork while holding it horizontally, approximately a foot from the ground, while the person at the base of the cock continued to pull out the handfuls of hay until eventually the sugán would be long enough to reach the opposite side where it would be tied around a long shaped stone to keep a weight on the cock, to prevent high winds from blowing off the tops. As well as the hayfork, a sickle (reaping hook) as it was called in Connemara could be used.

In my earliest memories of the hay being transported to the hayshed it was loaded on a horse and cart where the load had to be secured with ropes for the journey on the cart.

In later years each cock of hay was towed directly by placing a strong rope or chain around the base and hooked up to a horse's harness and towed to the hayshed.

We had a very large hayshed made of corrugated iron with the traditional curved roof and the sides and ends not reaching the ground to allow ventilation. When Bernard and myself got older we worked at storing and packing the hay into the shed. This was a strenuous task in warm weather but we enjoyed the satisfaction of having it fully saved and stored for the coming winter.

The Threshing

Growing cereals in Connemara was a very small item in farming and the most common cereal was oats, which was grown in small quantities in small fields. This was fed mostly to hens in most farms and occasionally to horses. There was no such thing as threshing mills. The small amount of threshing was carried out by an ancient method, which was very simple. A plank was placed on trestles with a big stone or more placed on the plank and one or two men would bash or thresh the head of the sheaf on the stone to beat out the grain, which fell on to sheets of tarpaulin where it would be collected for winnowing on a later date. This was carried out on a dry windy day by throwing the mixed grain and chaff on to a sheet of tarpaulin when the wind blows away the chaff and the heavier grain falls on the tarpaulin.

Summer

In the early thirties the roads had not been tarmacked. In the summer months I can remember the clouds of dust raised by the frequency of passing cars, mostly English holidaymakers. Connemara appeared to be a very popular area for tourists.

We frequently had our own relations visiting Ballyconneely. My aunt and uncle the Mathis's who had been in Marconi's Station had been posted to Egypt after the station closed down. They had two sons who were older than us and they were in a boarding school in England. They spent some of their summer holidays with us and they enjoyed the freedom and activities around the farm and swimming in the local beaches. Our cousins from Kerry also came on occasions. Our maiden Aunt, Kathleen, came on a long holiday from Hawaii every five or six years. She was the typical American and had very interesting stories of life and experiences on the pineapple and sugarcane plantations in Hawaii and of the long journey home by sea and land from Honolulu to Ballyconneely, which was a story in itself.

She found the Connemara climate very cold compared to the tropical heat in Hawaii but she still enjoyed her holiday and visited many old friends during her time at home, which was usually about four weeks.

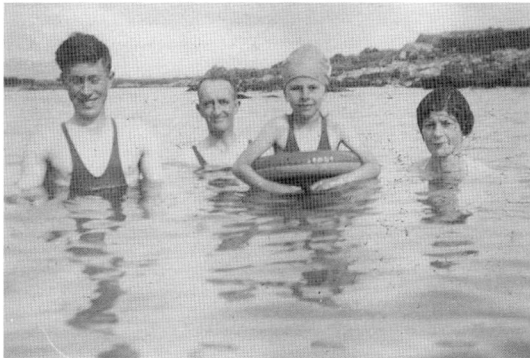

Bernard, Father, Carmel, Mother. Erriseask.(1942)

Pearl Harbour

She had a great mistrust of the large number of Japanese people in Honolulu and was convinced that they were up to no good. A few years later she was found correct as she was in Honolulu on the night of the 7th December 1941 when Pearl Harbour was bombed.

On the next day she sent a cablegram to Ballyconneely to reassure everybody that she was safe. When she was home on her last visit after the war she had the entire graphic details and description of that night of terror. She died in Waikiki in the late fifties. My wife Eileen and myself were on holidays there in 1985 but unfortunately we had mislaid her address so despite great efforts to trace her grave we did not succeed.

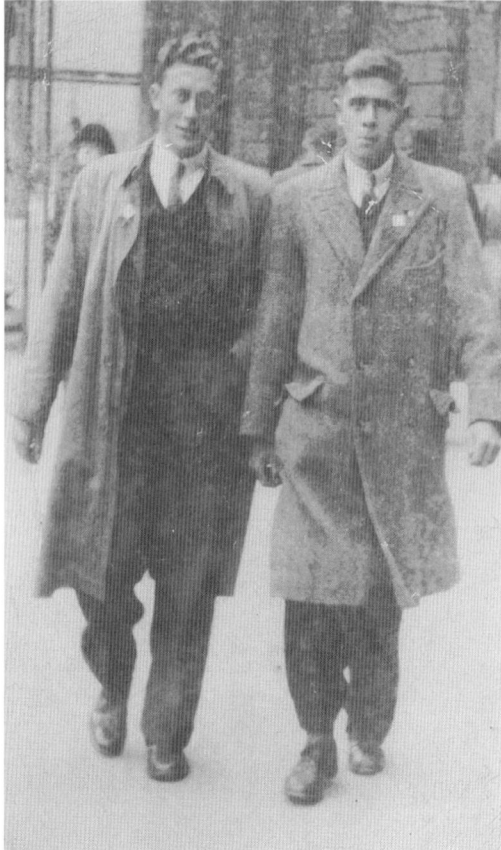

Ken, Bernard. Dublin.(1941)

Seaweed

There was another farming activity not as pleasant as the harvesting of the hay and turf, this was collecting and gathering up seaweed washed up on the sand by the sea. This was a well-known activity by farmers along the west coast who used the seaweed as a natural fertiliser for the land either on meadows or for crops particularly for potatoes.

There are several species of seaweed so the material washed up on the shore would contain a mixture of species and when left for a while on the sand it began to rot and gave out a mixture of odours.

The more decomposition that occurred, the better the quality. These deposits of seaweed were called wrack. In mid winter the wrack was gathered up and loaded on to a horse and cart and taken to a suitable site on the farmland and made into a large compost heap by mixing in ashes and turf mould (the original peat moss) and then left for several weeks before being transported once more to the bare meadows where it was left in small heaps all over the fields. These little mounds or heaps were then scattered around as finely as possible by men and children using pitchforks. We were still a long way from 'Muck spreaders' in those days.

This compost system was not usually used for the potato crop, for this, a particular type of seaweed was used. It had to be cut freshly from the rocks covered or partially covered by the sea during neap tides but exposed for a short time each day during spring tides.

The 'expedition' for this seaweed was an adventure for Bernard and myself to go on this apparently long trip in the horse and cart along the sandy beach to reach exposed rocks. The men then set to work cutting the seaweed with a reaping hook (sickle) while we went off knocking barnachs (Irish word for limpets) from the rocks to take home and to fry or roast them in their shells on the big range in the kitchen.

It was very important that men and children kept a close watch on the tide, which could surround them when the tide turned to come in (flow).

While we enjoyed all this activity we were always frozen with the cold and glad to be on the return journey home, which we had to walk as the cart or carts were now full. However, the walk soon heated us up.

This seaweed was later laid along the ground in the shape of a ridge and the seeds or slits of the potatoes placed in rows on top of the seaweed. The seed of the potatoes are one, two or three small 'eyes' that are visible on the potato. The potato is cut into

1 – 3 sections each containing an 'eye'. These sections were called slits in Connemara. With the slits in place the ridge was completed by a man digging up the scraw clay and placing it upside down on top of the seaweed. This system was used in the films, 'The Man of Aran' and 'The Field' but there was one big difference in 'Man of Aran' where there was only rock and some sand underneath a mixture of a little clay and sand on top.

As gardeners are aware tomatoes belong to the same horticultural family and for many years I used all kinds of seaweed collected along the shores of Lough Foyle for my own home grown tomatoes.

I did not use a horse and cart for transport but like the modern way of saving turf stuffed it into fertiliser bags, which I loaded into the boot of the car. For a few years, if there was no wrack or seaweed on the sand, I used the spring tide system and cut off fresh seaweed from nearby rocks with the reaping hook until one day a passer by informed me that this cutting from the rocks was now illegal. In addition to its uses for fertilising, seaweed was and still is used for industrial purposes and was harvested in the Ballyconneely area. My father was an agent for a company in Liverpool called 'The Borax Company' who processed the dried species of the material, which was called by its Irish name 'Caurlich'. This was harvested by local farmers from rocks covered or partially covered during neap tides and usually by boats during spring tides when the rocks became more exposed. Caurlich is a long very broad species, which can be seen, mixed with other species on the beach and is usually attached to a sea rod. When brought ashore the caurlich was then dried in the sun, sometimes with great difficulty in bad weather. When perfectly dry it was packed tightly into jute bags and stored in a big shed until a ship arrived to transport it to Liverpool. The packing and storing was all carried out on Bunowen Pier. The Limerick Steamship Company usually owned the ships used and the day she arrived was a big day in my eyes.

The blowing of the ship's hooters was the first sign of activity and this alerted local fishermen to bring one of their members out to board the ship to pilot her through the hazardous seas near Slyne Head. A large gang of local men would have assembled on the pier to carry the bags from the sheds on to the ship.

In addition to the caurlich, sea rods were also harvested then dried and burned in a type of kiln to form a semi-solid mass of a type of ash known as 'Kelp'. Both 'Kelp' and processed caurlich are used in chemical industries, the most notable being gelatine and cosmetics. The seaweed industry as I remember it was thriving up to the forties in Ballyconneely but like many other things changes occur. I have seen stacks of fresh seaweed along the roadside in recent times so I presume it is still used in industry.

Sea Fishing

In the Ballyconneely area and probably in many areas in the thirties white fishing could be classed as a cottage industry. The currach was the traditional boat and this was built by using light wooden laths as ribs to build the frame with a very sloping bow. This frame was then covered with a special canvas, which was treated and painted over with tar. There was another type of boat also called currachs. The only difference between the two was the latter had more wood and was heavier.

Individual fishermen would take a certain amount of fish to Clifden on the Friday, the traditional market day, when the fishermen loaded the fresh fish into creels on their horses and then mounted the horse to sit side-saddle behind the creels for the journey to Clifden. Large quantities of fish came to Clifden from the small islands on the north-west side of the town. Women mainly carried out the selling.

Lobster and crayfish fishing appeared to be more organised and possibly more lucrative for those involved. These fish appeared to have been very plentiful and certainly very much larger in size in those days than they are in modern times. They were caught in pots along the coast and were brought to the harbour in Bunowen where my father had them stored in large wooden tanks moored in the harbour and partially submerged.

When the tanks were full the lobsters were taken out and packed in sawdust in special boxes and then transported by train from Clifden to Dublin to some fish merchant for distribution to fish outlets. Lobsters could survive in sawdust for well over a day. When the railway closed in 1935 it was probably the end of the sawdust era. My memory is vague about some events at that time but I have a clearer memory of my father being an agent for a man in St. Malo, France. His name was Monsieur Samzun. At that time, when the tanks were full, the lobsters and crayfish were transferred to a natural sea pond in Aucharis near Claddaghduff, North West of Clifden. This large storage pond was formed by high rocks on three sides of an inlet with the open end controlled by a sluice gate which let the tide in and out but retained enough water at low tide to cover the lobsters. Eventually they were transferred to St. Malo on a ship with a special tank. Lobster and crayfish are still an industry in this area but are now a very special and expensive delicacy. In more modern times they were transported to Shannon and flown to France.

Bunowen

Bunowen is an historic area taking its name from the Irish 'Bun' meaning 'bottom or end', 'owen' meaning 'river'. There are numerous towns and areas all over Ireland situated at the mouth, bottom and end of rivers, big and small, and as a result are named 'Bun' this, that or the other (for instance where I have lived for 46 years, the local town Moville is called 'Bun an Phobail' as 'Bottom of the Foyle'.

There was an ancient castle in Bunowen near the end of the river, which was once owned by Granuaile where she lived for a short time with her then husband Dhonal Na Coga O'Flaithairte in English Dhonal of the Wars O'Flaherty (no relation).

As would be expected Dhonal was killed in a fight over territory. She then left the castle, which eventually fell into ruin and most of its stones were later used to build a more modern castle at the foot of Doonhill by the Blake's who were big landowners. Members of the Blake family used the castle as a summer residence. I accompanied my mother to afternoon tea there once. The inside was never completed and I thought it was really weird. This castle is still standing but roofless.

The Bar

As was the case everywhere in rural areas the bar was adjoined to the family home and the majority of the bars also had it combined with a grocery business. In Ballyconneely 'the bar' was a large square shaped area with a high 'bar' taking up two sides and the grocery with a low counter on the other side. There was also a built in Snug as was the custom in those days. The Snug was a small wooden structure with a door leading into it from the main bar. There was also a door leading on to the inside of the bar. There was a shelf and wooden seat on two sides acting as a mini bar on one side. The custom was that this area could be used by request for a small group of people who wished to have a private conversation or conduct business.

It was also used by small groups of ladies who wished to have a chat while drinking their sherry as in those days' ladies did not drink in the main bar. Inside the high bar there was a counter or shelf directly under the top of the 'high bar'.

This had a draining board and a sink for washing glasses. Attached was the machine with the big corkscrew for rapidly drawing corks from the stout and beer bottles. The only beer in existence then was 'Bass' and there was no such thing as an 'Iron Lung'. (The Iron Lung was a slang term for the iron barrel which came at a later date). In those days stout or porter was contained in the old wooden barrels which made 'Guinness' famous.

As we grew up we learned the technique of rolling the full barrels from the yard around a corner into the bar and then leaving it on its side on the ground or standing on one end to enable us to insert the heavy brass tap into the bung in the barrel. This was a special art to be carried out smoothly without creating a mess. The nozzle of the tap was wrapped up with a strip of brown paper to act as a sealer. With a steady hand the nozzle was held directly on the bung. A large wooden mallet was then held in the other hand with a steady grip and ensuring that the mallet head was not deviating to either side, then and only then, a fast heavy blow was aimed and came down on the end of the tap which should have sent the nozzle and bung cleanly and well into the barrel without any mess. If the mallet or tap had deviated in any way the brown froth would gush out and could go in any or all directions including hitting the ceiling. Needless to say my father rarely ever misfired and I can only remember attempting the job once and suffice to say it was not very successful! Bernard got it right from the start.

There was a special technique in lifting the full barrel on to the wooden stand without injuring one's back or bringing on a hernia. I am not going into the details of that. When the 'iron lung' was introduced, the stout was pumped up and powered by using a cylinder of oxygen or some other gas which was stored in a cellar.

Although I developed the skills of filling pints with good heads and serving the drinks, I never liked the drink culture.

I had no problem working on and off in the bar but I could never bring myself to understand how people could enjoy filling themselves and their friends with drink unnecessarily, almost amounting to force feeding, just to keep the 'round' system going. I could understand people enjoying moderate drinking at meal times at home or in restaurants or even in pubs but the race to force feed each other was and is totally beyond my comprehension. However I did see the positive side in that they were contributing to my future education.

When I was about ten years of age the Pioneer Total Abstinence (from alcohol) Association was in full swing. For an adult to become a member he or she had to be fourteen years of age and serve as a probationer for two years before becoming a full member. Different badges were worn to distinguish the grades. There was also a juvenile grade that could be joined at 12 years of age. At age ten I had decided that I would join the juvenile branch and I thought that the time would never arrive to show off my badge.

Naturally, living in a pub I had tasted several alcoholic drinks including stout, whiskey and sherry all of which I disliked. In those days when anybody had a high temperature from the Flu or sore throat whether adult or child they were given hot punch to drink at night. This consisted of whiskey in hot water, which I detested. I just hated the taste of it and I still have memories of my mother holding my nose with one hand and with the other hand pushing hot whiskey spoonful after spoonful into my mouth.

While it was horrible at the time I have been forever grateful to her for that forced feeding which put me off drink for life. Bernard also disliked the pub culture. He loved woodwork, fixing cars or anything that needed repairs and best of all farming. He did not become a total abstainer but enjoyed a very moderate drink. Carmel also disliked the drink culture but she also enjoyed a moderate drink.

My father appeared to enjoy the pub life and rarely got uptight when some drunk started messing and annoying everybody. When the occasional row started he went into the middle of it and could calm down the protagonists, without any fuss then he directed them to the door leaving most of them outside, then closed and locked the door and frequently put the shutters on the windows to make sure that nobody got pushed through a window. He was also a moderate drinker who enjoyed the occasional bottle of stout and a half one as the small measure of whiskey was called. My mother like most women of her time enjoyed the occasional glass of sherry. Wine was almost unheard of.

Dancing

At that time Ballroom Dancing was a feature in the famous Clifden Town Hall and were known as 'All Night' dances and that was all night, from 10pm to 3am and sometimes 4am. Special licences had to be obtained and there was a limit to a certain amount of these late dances per year.

These were on special occasion nights like Bank Holidays, Race Nights, The Garda Ball, and Show Night. In the thirties some of these dances also provided a late supper in the hall. There were several big dance bands around the west at that time. In my opinion the most famous and popular band was 'Stephen Garvey's Orchestra' who travelled from Castlebar fifty miles away. I am not sure when these dances became popular, probably in the late twenties, but as far back as I can remember our parents went frequently and enjoyed them. All the ladies wore evening dress and the men wore their best suits.

In the forties the older generation gradually bowed out and our generation gradually took over with 'Glen Miller Music', 'Joe Loss' etc.

There was another dancing system where there were many more short dances from 8-12 run by various clubs usually for fund raising, many of them were a mixture of céilí and old time dances.

Electric Power

Clifden had a local electric power supply generated by water from the local river, which flowed down a steep waterfall before entering the sea. This supply was there for many years before the ESB arrived in the early fifties.

There was no power in Ballyconneely except in the local Catholic Church where a very enterprising curate installed this in 1931-32 when he got the whole church refurbished including a very efficient lighting system. A local man George McWilliams who lived beside the church and looked after the running of the generator installed this. His family were our next-door neighbours and he lived with his mother who ran a grocery shop and his aunt was the postmistress. Bernard and George got on very well together at farming and fixing machinery.

Fair Days

Clifden, like numerous other towns and villages throughout the country had its monthly fair on a certain day every month and similar to many other places the fairs were held on the main street. There were also many places that had special fair greens.

Preparations for the fair began in Ballyconneely a day or two previously. When the best looking animals were picked out in the fields and brought to a semi-enclosed area near the house to be 'branded'. The customs in those days was that each farm had a metal brand usually in the shape of the initials of the owner so ours had a large OF, on the bottom of a long metal handle. The initials were dipped into a bucket of liquid tar and pressed on to the animal's hindquarter.

At around 6.30am on the morning of the fair two workmen got the cattle on the road and drove them the five miles to Clifden. My father went later in the car accompanied by Bernard and myself if we were off school.

Each farmer usually had a favourite area to herd the cattle but did not have a right to any particular place if it was already occupied. We usually got near the bottom of Market Street near our cousin's, the Lees, house. Two or three people with good hazel sticks kept the animals well controlled. Not a pleasant job on a wet cold day.

Bargaining between the owner and the jobber or cattle dealer, as they were also known carried out the selling transaction. Usually the jobber arrived into town the night before or the early morning. My memories of them were that they were all big men with red faces and wore heavy brown boots and felt hats and heavy twill or corduroy trousers.

The dealing was carried out by the long established method of the owner demanding an outrageous price and the jobber offering a ridiculously low price. As the agreement got closer there was frequent banging of the palms, spitting on palms and banter until eventually the deal was made and the jobber produced a tube of Raddle to mark each animal. The cattle pre 1935 were then driven to the railway station and post 1935 to cattle trucks.

By early afternoon the street would be awash with cattle dung while some shopkeepers were doing their best with hoses and buckets to wash it down the hill. Cattle were not always sold if a deal was not agreed so they would then drive them back home and wait until the next fair.

Eventually by the late fifties and sixties Marts sprung up very rapidly and the old fair day vanished to be replaced by weekly marts with cattle no longer driven miles along the roads but transported in smaller lots on tractors and trailers or in large lots on trucks.

Corpus Christi

During the thirties I remember the 'Corpus Christi' procession, which was a Catholic Church religious demonstration honouring the 'Body of Christ' in the 'Eucharist'. This took place once a year on a certain date after Easter, which was usually in June and traditionally from the Parish Church in Clifden. Large crowds from all over the parish gathered in the church and then went in procession, led by a priest holding up the Host in a Monstrance, and proceeded slowly around the town which would be brightly decorated with bunting across the main street and a small altar decorated with flowers at all doorways. The most popular flowers that I can remember were the rhododendrons, which invariably got blown down with the wind. Needless to say in our climate the day was frequently washed out by rain. This religious demonstration gradually disappeared with the onset of more traffic and also the progress of Ecumenism.

Altar Boys and Bell Ringers

On the subject of religion Bernard and myself for a few years before leaving school were altar boys. As the church door was only about thirty yards away we had no problems getting to the church on time. The altar boys carried out the chore of ringing the bell and this was a job enjoyed by all. It was a large bell high up in an open belfry with a long chain.

The more senior boys trained the new recruits on the finer arts of getting the rhythm correct between the ding and the dong as the chain went up and down. It was important not to pull while the bell was half way between the ding and the dong because if so you got no sound.

The bell ringing on New Year's Eve was carried out by young men probably experienced retired altar boys whose aim was to pull the bell out of the Belfry. The tradition was that the ringing out the old year began at ten minutes to midnight then there was a pause of one minute and then rang in the New Year for another ten minutes. Bernard and myself got in on the act for a few years. It was a great thrill as the chain was handed around to keep the ringing going at high pitch.

Breaking Stones and Roads

As far as I can recall tarmacking of the roads around Ballyconneely in the late thirties and that put an end to the clouds of dust raised by tourist cars during the summer months.

Before the work could begin stones had to be quarried and distributed along the roadsides for putting a new surface on the road.

The first task was to extract stones from nearby quarries and in those days this was a slow and dangerous work without the machines of later years. To get the stones out the rock had to be blasted to produce large stones, as there were no pneumatic drills so the holes for the gelignite had to be drilled by hand. This hole was approximately one foot deep and about an inch in diameter. Despite observing the procedure on a few occasions I cannot be precise about those measurements and I certainly was not around when the actual blasting was being carried out.

The drill was a heavy long bar, about three feet in length and an inch in diameter. It had a flat top and a bevelled bottom. Two men were required for the drilling; one grasped the drill with two hands and held it straight up on the spot to be drilled. The other man then struck the flat top part of the drill with a heavy blow of a sledgehammer. After one or two blows the man holding the drill rotated it slightly and continued this rotating after every one or two blows of the sledgehammers until the drill had gradually progressed down the hole to the required depth when the required numbers of holes were drilled the blasting operation was carried out by the ganger who prepared the gelignite to put it into the hole or holes and then attached it to a fuse then all workers or other people around were instructed to go for cover.

When the blast or blasts went off the ganger returned to the quarry to confirm if it was safe for everybody to return.

After blasting, the workmen, with crowbars and sledge hammers, broke up the blasted rock into stones which were then transported by horse and cart and distributed along the roadside to be broken into small stones by men using small hammers. These men were seated along the roadside. This was a very cold and boring task.

In modern times this work is carried out by one man or women in a cockpit of a huge machine like a steel dinosaur that can dig and break up stones by moving various levers. The stone crusher has replaced the man with a small hammer.

Even in the thirties there was one machine, which fascinated us, and that was the steamroller with its driver and helper. They did not live locally so they lived in the special caravan provided by the County Council. When they worked in Ballyconneely we got friendly with them and they invited us in to see the caravan.

It was winter so we were very impressed with the heat provided by the small stove, the bunk beds and general furnishings. The helper was also the cook so they provided us with tea and cake. One of them was a brilliant violinist so we enjoyed our visits immensely as there were also two other local men enjoying their hospitality and music. I am sure that the steamroller and caravan moved on after three or four days. We could have visited three times at most but it was a thrilling experience for two small boys that I have never forgotten.

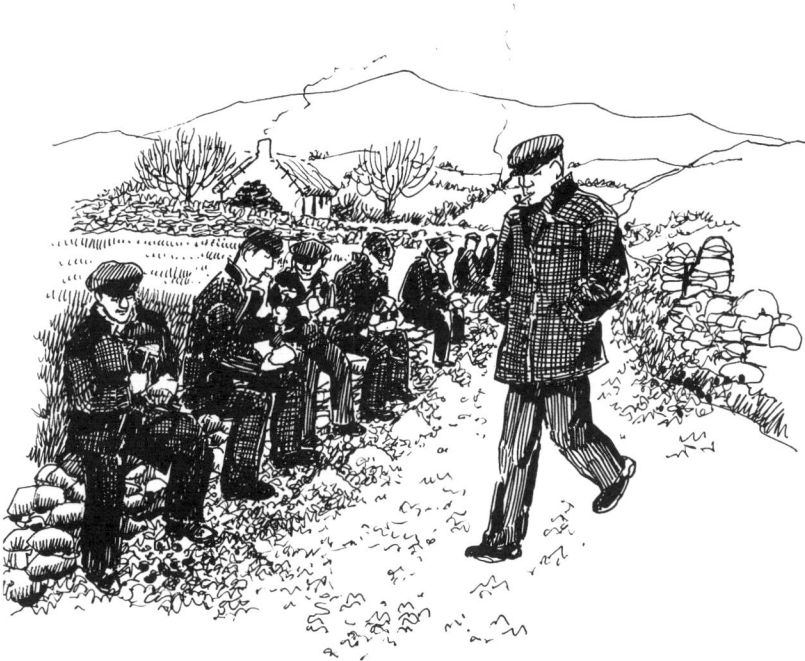

Wind and Water

This was another development that took place in the same era. There was no mains water supply in Ballyconneely in the thirties but in our house a private supply from rainwater collected in two cement tanks on a flat part of the roof. The house was a large two storey, part of it slated so that provided rainwater for the two tanks. These tanks provided a water supply for the bar and flush toilets and hot and cold water for baths. A back boiler in the kitchen range provided the hot water.

This system was adequate up to a point but the one drawback was the occasional dry summer when water had to be collected from the lake to fill barrels on a cart and pumped up from the barrels by a portable pump.

For some years my father and other local people had been trying to persuade the council to provide a waterworks.

Eventually inspecting various sources of an adequate water supply and carrying out water tests, it was decided to go ahead with a project. As there was no prospect of a gravity feed and no mains electricity available it was decided to use 'wind power' which was free of charge and in plentiful supply.

The lake selected for sourcing the water was a large deep lake part of which was touching on our land. The plan was to build a reservoir on high ground near the lake and use a large windmill to pump the water into it for filtering and distribution to a main pipeline along the main road so that a mains water supply was now available to households, public pumps and drinking troughs for cattle. This amenity reduced the drudgery of transporting water in barrels on horse and carts.

There were problems with the windmills being frequently damaged by storms but it was reasonably well maintained and I assume that when the E.S.B. arrived in the early fifties electric pumps would have been installed.

Wind Power

In the early forties wind power was tried for generating electricity for lighting individual houses. As people were becoming impatient waiting for electricity from the national grid and aggravated by scarcity of paraffin oil due to the war.

The system was that a single unit consisting of an iron stand secured in concrete and supporting a pole on top of which was a single propeller which charged a dynamo connected to a wire which carried power to the connections in the house.

Several of these wind chargers appeared around Connemara and my father had one installed in Ballyconneely. While it provided light it was erratic despite the fact that the propeller was fitted with a governor but it did help to spare the paraffin oil.

As we all know wind power has been used for generations around the world. But despite placing men on the moon and placing robots in various planets to collect samples and take photographs and then return to earth all by remote control, scientists have not yet really harnessed the wind. I believe this is due to inertia rather than lack of technology with fossil fuels running out and the earth becoming warmer. It is hard to believe that it is only in recent years that any real advance on the little wind chargers of sixty years ago has been made and what I believe is pathetic is the objections that are being made to the erection of modern wind generators.

The Forge

As we are still describing life and growing up in the thirties the forge must get special mention. I have no doubt that the forge and the blacksmith were always a great attraction for children growing up in small towns and villages.

In the early thirties there was no forge in Ballyconneely Village but there had been one in Ailbrack, which had closed down so an enterprising local man decided to train as a farrier and blacksmith and build a forge in Ballyconneely.

His plans were successful and in due course the forge was built a very short distance from our house where the main road veered off to Roundstone and a by-road continued on to Ailbrack and Bunowen.

Between the forge and the house there was a semi-circular wall just off the road which had a number of iron rings secured in a dangling position along the wall. These rings were used for tying horses and donkeys when the owners were shopping or drinking. The wall was always kept whitewashed and we always referred to it as 'The Rings'.

Shoeing

We frequently visited the forge and enjoyed watching the blacksmith at work and were amazed at his skill and speed in heating the iron for the horseshoes to a red hot heat in the fire by holding the iron in tongs with one hand and operating the big bellows with the other hand, pulling a wooden shaft up and down, then shaping the pliable hot iron with a hammer at great speed on the anvil. When the shoe began cooling it was then pressed on the horses hoof to check how well it fits and usually with slight re-heating and more work on the anvil gets the correct size, which is then nailed on to the hoof with special horseshoe nails.

The Cartwheel

Horses and donkeys was the farrier part of the job, the blacksmith part entailed making iron gates and numerous other iron objects and tools, which involved another specialist skill and that was 'shoeing' cartwheels. A cartwheel was made of wood and iron tyres or rims. The wheel was made up of several slightly curved sections of wood called 'Felloes'. When all were joined together end to end they formed a circle into which one end of each spoke was inserted. The other end was inserted into the hub or heart of the wheel, which was cylindrical shaped block of wood, which encased the axle in a hollow metal casing.

The iron tyre would start as a long rod of iron the same width as the wheel rim. The iron was then curved by the blacksmiths to roughly fit the wheel, which was now placed, on a concrete base with a circular hole placed in the centre to take the heart of the wheel and keep the rest of the wheel steady.

The next step was to build a circular turf fire on and around the circular iron a little distance from the waiting wheel.

When the iron was almost red hot it was lifted by at least three men using special tongs and carried the short distance to the wheel and hammered down quickly while buckets of water were very quickly doused over it to prevent too much burning.

The old type blacksmith has now passed into a history but the Farrier part has become a highly trained specialist for shoeing thoroughbred racehorses, show jumpers and all types of ponies. The blacksmith part has become the highly trained welder who works with acetylene gas instead of coal, smoke and dust.

Errismore

'Erris' is the Irish word for' Peninsula' and 'mor' is the word for 'big or large'.

Joyce said that a pier was a frustrated bridge so it could be fair to say that a peninsula was a frustrated island.

South of Clifden, there are three peninsulas all off which add to the beauty and wilderness of West Connemara. The most northerly is Errislannin called after the local Saint Flannin who must have come from Clare. It is situated between Clifden Bay on the north and Mannin Bay to the south.

Errismore, the big Peninsula is situated between Mannin Bay and Ballyconneely Bay. 'Errisbeg' the 'Small Peninsula' is situated between Ballyconneely and Roundstone. Errismore stretches from Derrygimla to Slyne Head and has its own striking beauty spots. The road from Clifden to Ballyconneely skirts the famous coral sands where there is a coarse type of sand resembling coral.

This coral sand is literally beside the road just a few steps from a car or bicycle to the sands, which gradually merge with fine silver strands stretching away towards Mannin Beach.

The road continues through Ballyconneely Village on to Bunowen pier and Ailbrack where the Connemara Championship Golf Links is situated. From there it is possible to walk to Slak Port and on to Ballinleim where in the era of the manned lighthouses the light keepers travelled by open boat in the hazardous seas to Slyne Head when the weather was favourable. Frequently due to bad weather several days or even weeks could delay the relief.

Slyne Head Lighthouse was built on the largest of the small islands in the area in the early part of the nineteenth century. A short time later another lighthouse was built which was closed down later so this makes Slyne Head unique in having two towers and one light.

Saint Cauline the Patron Saint of Errismore was reputed to have had a religious establishment in the Slakport area and as with all local saints he had a holy well which is still a place of pilgrimage on the 13th November, which is a landmark day for the coming of Christmas as it is exactly six weeks before Christmas Day. I am not that very sure of this but he was reputed to have been a brother of St Flannin.

As in most parts of the country, flapper horse racing was, and still is, a great sport and social occasion during the summer months. Errismore was no exception. In the

Clifden area there were four meetings. The Clifden Races were always held on the August Bank Holiday on a racecourse called 'Curvaghal' is now a large holiday home complex, known as 'Clifden Glen'. There was also a meeting in Omey Island north of Clifden. The actual races were held on the big strand during a low tide.

This was a beautiful setting for a race meeting but the date of the event and the time of racing were dependent on the tides. There was a meeting in Lettergesh also held on a magnificent strand near Renvyle which was used for a race scene in the 'Quiet Man' film in 1951.

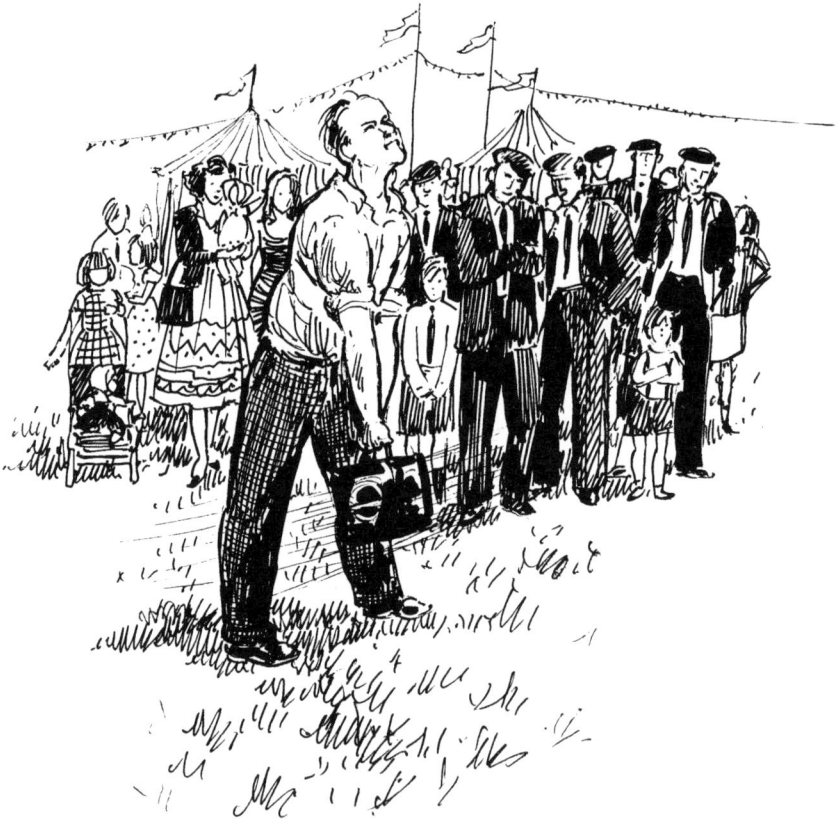

Errismore Races

The Errismore races were reputed to be the oldest race meeting in Connemara, first held in 1898, but I have no doubt that claim would be contested. The races were held on different dates in August on the magnificent beach in Alibrack in the area south west of the golf course.

The eve of the race day was usually exciting for Bernard and myself as a horse owner north from Clifden used to stable his racehorse in one of our carthorse stables on the evening before the races. We were intrigued watching the groom brushing the horse, feeding it with special clean non-musty hay and some oats. In those days licensed bars were permitted at race meetings so usually a publican from Clifden would set up a temporary bar in the open air.

This was carried out by long boards on trestles to form a square counter, which would be a hive of activity for the duration of the meeting.

There were all the other usual stalls, roulette, the airgun target shooting, the ice cream van, the three card trick man who always won and his counterpart the man with the upturned empty tin box and elusive nut. Last but not least was the loveable settled traveller from Clifden with the black and white chequered square of lino who invited competitors to land a penny on certain squares to win a small amount of pennies.

To attract the punters he had a famous cry which could be heard at a distance and went like this 'Hump-them-dump them-any way you like, you'll up to the bank in the morning'.

The setting of this course was perfect for racing. It was a hard sandy and grassy beach with an extensive flat area and also a raised rocky area for viewing and picnics with a glorious view very close to the sea and beautiful silver strand.

In addition to the horses and the side shows there were also some athletic events like long and short distance running for adults and sprints for under fourteens and sixteens, also weightlifting for strong men. It could be said that this weightlifting was a native sport in Errismore. This sport involved using a 56lb weight with a strong rope tied around the lifting bar. The competitor lifted the weight by the rope and after dangling it back and forward between his legs, heaved it forward to make his mark wherever it landed. Bernard and myself had an interest in the sprints and frequently finished in the top three driven by the fact that all the prizes were cash. As far as I can remember the first prize was seven shillings and six pence, second prize was five shillings and third two shillings and six pence (the old half-crown). We could be classed as the first Professional Athletes.

My father was the race judge so he had to be available all during the meeting and frequently had to sort out disputes about close finishes, as there were no photo finishes available in those days.

When the races ended the day was not over as we had to rush back to the bar which was always very busy until closing time.

Swimming, Bonfires and Cornflakes

With all the activities in the summer months working at turf and hay and thinning turnips and rounding up cattle etc we still made time for swimming during the odd fine spells. As there was an abundance of beautiful sandy beaches we were spoiled for choice. In the long summer days we would go for a swim in the evening after working at hay or some other chore all day. We usually went to 'Erriseask' beach which was the nearest. My father would take the car to a short distance from the sea. More frequently we walked through the fields and on other occasions, cycled. There was another less sheltered beach where the car could be driven on to the sand when we required a quick swim. We rarely swam in the coral beach, as the water there was much colder.

My father was a good swimmer and taught Bernard, Carmel and myself a sort of basic breaststroke, which we stuck with for the rest of our lives and could, enjoy a swim in the sea or a pool any time we wished. My mother never learned to swim but she loved bathing and plunging up and down in the water and sun bathing.

On a very fine Sunday during the rare hot spells we all went for a picnic on Erriseask beach.

Now I wish to reassure the reader that we did not have a Mediterranean climate in Ballyconneely, far from it.

When I write about picnics it means probably an average of one every two years but they were the days when the photographs were taken and they were days we always remember.

There was another activity or tradition in the thirties and forties which was enjoyed by young and old and this was Bonfire Night or to put it more correctly 'St John's Night' the 23rd of June the eve of the Feast of St John. It was celebrated in pagan times to honour mid-summer. For several weeks before the event both young and old collected wood and all sorts of rubbish and lumps of bog oak, deal and heaps of turf and bushes which were placed on a big rock on raised ground.

When we were young children my father used to get us up late on that night to an upstairs window to see the vast number of bonfires springing up all around the countryside. Adults and children gathered around the fire and frequently had singing and music.

As we grew older we had our own bonfire for several years and I remember one night in particular when an adult with an accordion played well into a balmy morning.

It is sad that this great tradition appears to be dying out or dead but I am sure like the Wren boys it will be revived. I had always assumed that St. John's night was only celebrated in Ireland until (going fast forward) twenty three years later while on holiday with my wife Eileen in Norway. We were staying in a beautiful small resort called Ulvik on the Hardanger Fiord. By a huge coincidence we were there on the 23rd of June and were invited to go to the local celebration that night of 'En-Ion' or 'St. John'. We were informed that this was a big national celebration of St. John and mid-summer.

Their tradition was that the family had a big meal at home in the evening and then went to the bonfires at midnight where there is no real darkness and continued their celebration with music, singing and dancing.

On that memorable night they put on a magnificent show for tourists. They displayed their native dress, dancing and singing.

They all gave a brilliant display of the nation's national trolls who are mythical Scandinavian giants and dwarfs who live in caves somewhat like our fairies. That was our last night in Ulvik so we departed the next morning with great memories of the Hardanger Fiord and St. John's night in Ulvik.

Returning to my memories of the thirties there is another sad loss to our countryside and that is the virtual disappearance of our early summer friends – the corncrake and the cuckoo. While there are great efforts to save them I am sincerely hoping that they are not gone to join the Dodo. There appeared to be several corncrakes in the long grass near our house in Ballyconneely and they croaked continually all night.

The last time I heard one was during the day in Rossnowlagh in Co Donegal in 1982.

The Light Keepers

 Slyne Head being a rock station the light keepers had a system of duty with three men on duty for a certain number of weeks until relieved by another three keepers. The married men with families lived in special dwellings in Clifden when off duty. When relief time came the keepers were transported by hackney from Clifden to Ailbrack and this also included each man having a supply of provisions for his term of duty.

These provisions were contained in large hampers, which appeared to be wrapped in a black waterproof material to protect them from the rain and high seas between the mainland and the island.

The keepers frequently called into Ballyconneely to have some light refreshment and a chat with my father before resuming duty or returning to Clifden for a well earned break.

From a very young age I became very familiar with the comings and goings of the light keepers and as I will record later this association lasted until Eugene O'Sullivan Junior the last man to leave the service departed from Howth Lighthouse in 1990. Returning to the relief system – when the hackney car reached the end of the road at Ailbrack Beach, the supplies and men were loaded on to a horse and cart which transported them to the contractors house (the King's in Slak Port) which was the last house on the mainland and the luggage was then transferred to donkeys until reaching the slipway in Ballinleim, then, on to the boat for the hazardous journey to the lighthouse. The journey sounds like the 'Odyssey of Ulysses' but I have no doubt but there were many similar journeys around the coast before the helicopters arrived. Slyne Head was de-manned and automated in 1990 the same year as I retired. I made one memorable trip to Slyne Head on a scorching hot summer's day sometime in the forties. I accompanied Bernard who was going there with a farmer to do a deal about buying sheep that the farmer had grazing on the island. It was a very pleasant trip, which included a tour of the lighthouse.

Returning to the thirties some of the light keepers were friendly with my uncle in Clifden. One of their men had the age-old light keeper's hobby of manoeuvring models of ships and crucifixion scenes into bottles. He had presented two of these models, one of a sailing ship and the other a crucifixion scene to my uncle.

When Bernard saw these, his first reaction was to state that he could do the same. The boat was put into a flat whiskey bottle and the crucifixion into a five naggin whiskey bottle.

Bernard decided to do the crucifixion scene in the long five naggin bottle so he started the job and after a few minor hitches he carved out all the parts with a pen knife on ordinary deal wood.

Having rehearsed assembling the parts outside the bottle, the next step was to repeat the procedure inside the bottle. Before taking this final step the inside of the bottle had to be sterilised thoroughly to kill any fungi or other contaminants so that when the sterilised water fills the bottle it will stay crystal clear. When he commenced the final assembly this was where I came in to hold the bottle steady while the assembly was being carried out successfully. Then the final act was to pour in the sterile water to soak the wood and to bind all the loose parts in their proper places. When the water-cooled the sterile cork was inserted and the job was done. He did two of them, one is still in his family home and I have the other, which is still intact and in perfect condition after sixty-three years.

Galway and The Men of Aran

Galway is situated fifty-five miles from Ballyconneely and in the thirties it appeared to be a very long journey by car for those fortunate enough to possess one. My father had a motor bike long before he was married, probably 1916 –20 and he then progressed to owning a model-T Ford which was eventually converted to a small truck and that was the first mode of transport that I can remember. In 1931 he purchased a 14.9 Ford Green Saloon car with a manual sliding roof (sunshine). It appeared to be a reasonably sized car.

The next car was the famous Baby Ford, which lasted for many years. We had very many journeys in both cars to Galway over the years. My father went frequently on business trips so mother, Bernard and I would be taken on many occasions.

The journey always appeared to be very long and in the wintertime very cold. The road was narrow and had numerous bends and hills.

Around that time the road was being surfaced and tarmacked. The journey took over two hours and despite the rugs and gloves, scarves and overcoats we were still frozen stiff when we arrived in Galway.

It now boggles the mind to try and believe that heating cars did not become standard until the nineteen sixties while the minimum technology was available from at least 1930's. When I purchased my first, new car, a Ford Anglia, in 1957 (the second half of the twentieth century) there was an option on having a heater fitted for twelve pounds and ten shillings extra, which I was delighted to pay. If the Japanese had not come on the scene we still would not have standard heaters or rear window wipers.
Returning to the trips to Galway it would be an early morning start on the road for the first five miles to Clifden to get to the main Galway road, which is a wonderful scenic journey. On leaving Clifden and reaching the right angle turn to the left at Waterloo Bridge (now gone) then past the racecourse area and now Clifden Glen Holiday Complex then on to Derrylea Lake which stretches alongside the road for the length of the lake. From there we rapidly approached Ben Lettery, the first of the twelve Bens, which overlook Ballinahinch Lake and castle. This lake has a small island on which there is the ruin of the ancient castle reputed to have been a stronghold of the O'Flaherty Clan (no relation).

There is a traditional story or legend that this little castle contained a trap door through which the owner presumably (Dhonal na Coga) disposed of his enemies into the lake. The road continues on to pass by the old Recess Railway Station. A road here leads through the mountains of the Joyce country to Gleninagh and Kylemore. In this area around Recess the world-renowned Connermara Marble is quarried.

The road then goes on to Maam Cross which once consisted of a pub and petrol pump, owned by a family by the name of Peacock, and served as a half way house between Clifden and Galway. It is now a very large establishment and tourist attraction. A road to the north leads to the Maam Valley, Leenane and Clonbur while the road to the south to Screebe and Rossavele.

The road is now leaving the mountains behind and going on towards Oughterard which has a beautiful approach where for a short distance the road goes alongside a tree-lined, fast flowing river.

The town being situated near the shores of Lough Corrib is a world renowned fishing centre and this becomes obvious as you enter the town by the number of long established hotels on each side of the main street, which appears to stretch for a long distance from one end of the town to the other end leading on to a tree lined road leaving the town towards Galway. The scenic humped bridge of Rosscahill soon comes into view where there was yet another scene of 'The Quiet Man'. We soon reach Moycullen, the nearest small town to Galway city; over these last few miles we usually passed several men with horses and cartloads of turf on their way to Galway to be sold to householders around the city.

I was always intrigued by the way the loads of turf were built on these carts compared to the Ballyconneely system where a rectangular crate three feet high was fastened on the body of the cart and when loaded the turf was built up slightly above the crate.

In Moycullen the turf appeared to be built from the body of the cart forming a pyramid supported by long sticks or laths tied around this high pyramid of turf. I always wondered how long it took to build this work of art.

Some of our trips to Galway involved visiting the dentist to have teeth filled which in those days was a prolonged and painful procedure.

On leaving Moycullen and overtaking all the turf carts the moment of truth was coming closer by the minute so the butterflies got busy up and down my back. Our dentist was Mr. Henry Anderson who had his surgery in Eglinton Street opposite the Savoy Cinema and which became the C.A.O. Office in later years.

He had played rugby for Ireland and he had photographs of the Irish teams on the waiting room walls. I had never seen a rugby match at that stage but frequently listened to commentaries of the Triple Crown Internationals so that raised him to hero status in my mind and may have helped to reduce the torture of the old filling drills. In later years he had the honour of being President of the Irish Rugby Football Union (I.R.F.U.).

On reaching the city, the car was parked in Eyre Square where there was usually a calf fair in progress and we would then proceed to the nearby Imperial Hotel for refreshment and to stretch our legs and in winter to thaw out having sat for fifty-five miles in our icebox.

On many occasions we saw the Aran men around the city in their traditional dress. They all appeared to be very big men in their wonderful native attire with the 'Tam O'Shanter' type woollen cap, either red or white, the Báineen jacket, the renowned Aran gansey (jumper/sweater), white or grey, and the homespun tweed trousers usually grey.

Many wore pampooties, a type of shoe, which were probably made from sealskins and the attire was completed with the red and white trouser belt known as the crios.
In those days the Aran people travelled on a historic boat that went from Galway docks to Aran. This was the 'Doon Aengus' and she carried passengers and cattle. The Aran people would also use the 'Galway Hooker', which was a sailboat that also carried turf to Aran. If mother was with us she went off to drapery shops and my father went to various business places, shops or wholesale establishments.

Usually the first visit was to McDonagh's the big wholesale place for fertilisers, hardware of every description including timber, iron, and farm implements etc. These premises were situated in the Claddagh area. He then visited a man who lived in Claddagh and sold jute bags, which my father required for storing Caurlich. This man had the bags stored in one of the great historic landmarks of Galway – the Spanish Arch (or Arches) which were part of the ancient City Walls and for all these years I wondered why the site was called the Spanish Arch not Arches and I also wondered why one of the Arches was used as a store and presumably why was such a historic 'Arch' in the old wall built up on one end? This year 2001 I discovered this opening in the wall was always called 'The Blind Arch', so I have at last got an explanation after sixty years why the Claddagh man was allowed to store bags in the blind arch (with a door on). McDonagh's very large premises were moved to a large site outside the city and Jury Hotels purchased the Claddagh site to build the Galway Jury Inn. The year it opened, Eileen and myself unknowingly booked for a weekend to the site where sixty years ago as a small boy I wandered around the big shop and stores and as our room was directly opposite the Spanish Arch and its blind companion and in that year 1997 I was still wondering about the man storing his bags.

Naughtons in Shop St was a very large retail hardware shop and appeared to have everything. It oozed a pleasant fresh scent of jute bags filled with seeds and with the bags opened for display. It had garden equipment of every description from large lawn mowers to small hand trowels, hedge clippers, spades and shovels of all sizes etc. In those days all large shops and stores had a special type of system for billing and change but Naughtons appeared to have a large system, which always got my attention when I was there.

In this system the salesman or woman put the customer's cash and bill into what appeared to be a hollowed wooden ball made up by two interlocking hemispheres to form a wooden ball. This sphere or ball loaded with cash and bills was shot up along a tubular frame by a hard pull on a string. It then landed on a semi-circular track suspended from the ceiling and sloped towards a cashier in the kiosk who sorted out the cash and receipt, stuffed it into the sphere and sent it back on another track going in the opposite direction or was it? The same track tilted towards the salesman (I think there were two). This system of long ago always fascinated me and I enjoyed watching the busy balls rolling hither and thither around the shop and it all appeared to me to be very efficient. Nowadays I can only see the salesperson touching buttons or tapping a square glass in a frame with a finger tip and a receipt pops up or pops out from the top or the side or the bottom of the little glass frame.

In the thirties, Galway had no Woolworths but they had Glyns which was the nearest thing and always worth a visit.

O'Gorman's Paper and Bookshop was the first place that I enjoyed that fresh scent of newly printed papers and books and gave me a lifetime pleasant addiction for browsing around bookshops.

The main reason for the visit in the thirties was to purchase comics usually the 'Beano' and 'The Dandy'. Bernard being older than me was more sophisticated and went for the 'Hotspur', which had more reading and stories about football. O'Gorman's has gone but fortunately has been replaced by Eason's.

Having described the various scents and aromas of several shops around Galway we have now reached the mother of all pleasant aromas that assails us as we approach Lydens Restaurant and Bakery from any direction that is the most wonderful aroma of all sorts of cakes, cookies, pastries, rolls, pancakes etc etc.

If proceeding to the restaurant a climax was reached when passing alongside the counter before ascending the stairs and as we ascend the winding staircase to the restaurant the experience gradually changes to the aroma of fresh cooking.

The waitresses wore dark green uniforms with white lace headbands and they were all very pleasant. The food was delivered from the kitchens on a small lift, which I cannot remember whether it descended from upstairs or ascended from downstairs but it was always good. The restaurant changed over the years and with the rapidly changing times and diets Lydens disappeared.

During the thirties aviation was developing rapidly and air displays were held in various venues around the country. In 1935 there was a display held in Oranmore just outside the city and air trips from there to around the city and part of Galway Bay were part of the show. My father was keen on flying and took Bernard and myself for a trip, which as far as I can remember was ten shillings each. My father enjoyed it immensely, Bernard also enjoyed it but I was terrified.

On our many journeys to Galway we had one minor accident, which appeared serious when it occurred. Somewhere between Moycullen and Oughterard, at night, when we ran into stray cattle on the road and killed a bullock and wrecked the radiator of the car. It took some time to carry out the usual necessary sorting out and then obtaining a hackney car to take us home, which we reached in the early hours of the morning.

The Connemara Pony and Shows

The Connemara pony is now renowned around the horse world for their beauty and resilience. I first heard of this type of horse as far back as I can remember. At that time in the early thirties they were not famous but there were a few very dedicated people who were determined to revive this breed. My father was not involved in this but he had a great interest in this revival, as he was a close friend of one of those people, Josie Mongan, who was involved.

It was thought that a breed of small ponies existed in ancient times and it was thought that they came to Ireland from the wrecks of the Spanish Armada but it was considered more likely that they may have come on some of the many Spanish merchant ships that traded between Spain and Galway

In 1923 the The Connemara Pony Society was founded and this led to the founding of the Connemara Pony Show, which gradually became a world-renowned show. The venues of the original shows alternated between Oughterard, Clifden, Roundstone and Carna.

For many years the show included cattle and sheep and home products and crafts.
I remember my father exhibiting cattle at the Clifden show on a few occasions when Bernard and myself were showing calves on halters and on one occasion awarded second and third prizes. Mother was very keen on shows and exhibiting jams. When the show was held several years in Carna she loved to travel the long distance to the venue. Since 1947 the show has a permanent base in Clifden on a site owned by the society and held every year in August where it attracts huge attendances from all over Ireland and also many visitors from the U.S. and Europe.

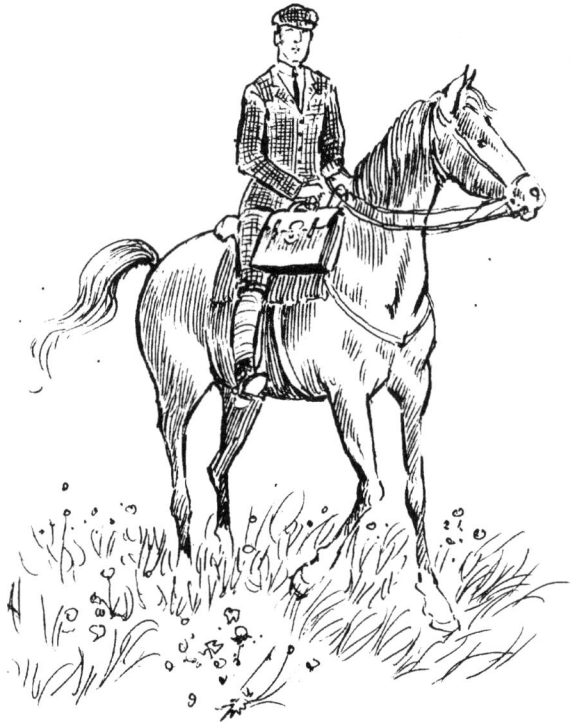

Education

All through our National School days all three of us had been well briefed by our mother on the importance of 'Learning our Lessons' (in recent times as I frantically refer to a dictionary I remember that she was 'a Devil' for the spellings) reminding us that we were very lucky to eventually be going to a boarding school.

As Carmel was eight and a half years younger than me she would have got the briefing much later. Bernard and myself had no problems about this and in fact looked forward to the day when we would go. Our parents, uncles, aunts and cousins had all been to boarding schools.

We frequently discussed the change but were not talking about study. It was always about the great-organised sport facilities that boarding school provided. During summer holidays we had seen older boys who were at boarding schools competing in athletics and playing football in their college colours. One thing we never had were football jerseys or shorts, we were lucky to have real football boots of which we took great care. Sport equipment was not available for young people at home in those days. Boys and girls who were at boarding schools were looked upon as 'heroes' or 'heroines' when they returned home on holidays.

There was no such thing as coming home at weekends or once a month. A school term was being there for every day of it.

While sport was our main concern we were well aware of the other side like corporal punishment, starvation, washing in ice-cold water, numerous rules and regulations, classes and study. All this was well worth it when the tog-out bell rang.

As we were approaching the end of our national school days, it had not been decided when and where to go but a decision must have been imminent.

Holidays and War

In a rural seaside area, holidays away from home were not necessary but for some reason in August 1939, all three of us with a lady who was a live in helper plus Laddie, the dog, were all sent on holiday to a rented cottage in Ashford, Co Wicklow. As the holiday was going to extend into September, boarding school was off the agenda for that year.

The holiday was a real novelty because we were away from the sea and in a wooded area with better land and much larger farms than in Connemara and for the first time we saw a large threshing mill working. We also saw a machine cutting a large field of wheat or barley. All these experiences were a real education, which we enjoyed.

On Friday 1st September we went on a trip to Wicklow Town and while there we heard a radio announcing that Hilter had bombed Danzig and had invaded Poland so that was the start of World War 2.

The official start came on Sunday 3rd September when the English Prime Minister Neville Chamberlain officially declared war on Germany.

That Sunday is also remembered, as the day of the 'Thunder and Lighting Hurling Final', between Cork and Kilkenny, in Croke Park when the whole match was played in a violent thunderstorm.

Two weeks later we were on our way home but first we were brought to see our first All Ireland Football Final in Croke Park between Meath and Kerry.

That morning we were brought to see our Aunt Agnes known as 'Archie'. At that time she was living in Dublin in Home Farm Road, Drumcondra.

She had three daughters, Harriet (Harry), Maureen and Muriel and one son Johnnie. The three girls were at school and college in Dublin and Johnnie worked with his father in their business in Dingle, Co Kerry.

While visiting Archie she brought up the subject of boarding school and as no arrangements had been made about us she very strongly recommended the school that Johnnie had been in and that he had been very happy there and most important was that the college had its own big farm and produced most of their own food. This was called Castleknock College situated beside the Phoenix Park in Dublin. The decision was then made that application would be made for us to start there the following year. That day Johnnie brought us to Croke Park to see the famous ground and the first of many All Ireland finals. This one was won by Kerry defeating Meath.

From Slyne Head to Malin Head, A Rural GP Remembers.

We returned to Ballyconneely the next day and then back to the National School for the last year. The war was now on but there were no dramatic changes in Ireland as the government had agreed that Ireland would remain neutral. Around that time a passenger liner was torpedoed off the west coast and many of the survivors were brought into Galway. This reminded everybody that the war had really started and it was accepted that the war would last a long time if it was to be similar to the 1914 to 1918 war.

Preparations for rationings were being made; this would include petrol, paraffin, coal, and other fuels, building materials and certain foodstuffs.

When the threat of war was looking inevitable my father hoarded a good supply of petrol in the garden shed, which was well out of reach of stores and dwellings if it blew up or caught fire. It lasted a long time until all private cars were put off the roads. Scarcity of solid fuel was not a problem in Connemara as coal was rarely ever used and there was always a plentiful supply of turf.

In actual fact turf became an industry during the war to supply Dublin and many other towns and areas away from bogs. This situation provided very welcome employment – the amount of turf supplied to Dublin must have been massive as I remember seeing the gigantic stacks of turf along the wide roads of the Phoenix Park until the early fifties.

Unfortunately, probably due to bad weather rushed harvesting and bad mossy bogs being used much of the turf reaching Dublin was of very poor quality as it always appeared to be wet. That type of turf in Connemara was known as 'Spartuch'. It was useless. I had personal experience of this attempting to light a much-needed fire in a digs in Dublin during the 1947 Freeze Up.

Returning to rationing of food, the scarcity of one commodity that caused the most distress to customers in Ballyconneely, and presumably elsewhere, was tea. Great efforts were made by various experts to produce a substitute beverage and eventually produced a drink called Coff O'Era. The customers called it by other names, which cannot be repeated here. In those days coffee was rarely used in Connemara.

In the early days of the war the government set up a coast watching service, which involved recruiting local volunteers who were given a basic training by army officers. Their function was to report any sightings of naval ships or any other such movement. Two men at a time were posted on top of coastal hills all around the country. A small hut was provided for shelter and powerful binoculars provided. As phones were very rare in all rural areas at that time special lines were installed to connect each watch post to the nearest post office.

The lookout post in Errismore was situated on top of Doon Hill in Bunowen. In very fine weather Bernard and myself occasionally visited the post to get the brilliant views on the powerful binoculars.

After the initial shock after the declaration of war, life went on normally in Ireland. Apart from the frequent reminders like news of merchant ships being sunk, frequently as a result of this large quantities of timber were being washed ashore along the west coast and Errismore was no exception particularly, south of Slyne Head. The wreckage was legally the property of the customs and excise but the quantities were so large that it was collected in all directions.

The Phoney War

On the declaration of war England did not have a large army or air force so they hastily sent a force called 'The British Expeditionary Force' to France to confront the German army. From that time until the spring of 1940 there was little or no fighting and this period was later known as 'the phoney war' but in the spring 1940 the real war was started and the Germans beat the British force back to the French Coast where the dramatic evacuation of Dunkirk took place in May. The real war had now started and an invasion of Britain became a real possibility and there was no doubt that this would include invading Ireland. The government ordered that all possible landing places along the coast were to be protected by digging small trenches over vast areas of seaside beaches. This was achieved by voluntary labour on the large expanse of Alibrack Beach, which was carried out using spades and shovels.

The L.S.F.

The local security force was then formed and this became known as the L.S.F. This involved local volunteers who would carry on their normal work at home but would go out in small groups at night to patrol local areas and to report any suspicious movements that would indicate possible or imminent invasion. My father was a member of this force. A similar force in England gave rise many years later to the famous TV comedy series 'Dad's Army'.

As the war went on another force for younger volunteers was formed and this became the Local Defence Force, which had full military training and is still in existence as a reserve army force. When Bernard finished school he joined and was a member for some years.

Around this time the infamous German Propaganda broadcaster known as 'Lord Haw Haw' came on the air and for a long time was threatening imminent invasion of Ireland. As he originally came from Galway he had a great knowledge of Irish geography. London and other parts of Britain were being bombed every night and this period became known as 'The Blitz'.

The early part of that summer was very intense and I thought that there would be no boarding school in September and that the country could be invaded and taken over by Hitler
.

As the summer moved on the threat of invasion appeared to be gradually receding so everybody became more relaxed and the big step to boarding school went on.

Castleknock

We had read the prospectus several times and were very impressed by the photographs of rugby and athletics teams but slightly disappointed that there was no mention of Gaelic teams.

My father drove us up and arrived there in the afternoon and was thrilled to see the grounds and the numerous goal posts around the place and also two full size handball alleys and a swimming pool.

There had to be something drastically wrong if we could not settle into this sort of life with the rules and regulations such as being confined to the grounds at all times except when permitted to go out. A day out was allowed once a month provided we had a letter from our parents.

Priests, The Vincentian Fathers, with some lay teachers, ran the college. The first few days were very relaxed settling in to new classes, then there was a religious Retreat which went on from Thursday night until Sunday morning in complete silence attending various religious services. When it ended after Grace before breakfast there was an almighty roar.

The College had a cinema projector, which had been presented to them by a past student. This projector was operated by one of the priests. There was a cinema show once a month and on 'free days', which were usually, feast days of Vincentian Saints. The shows took place in the recreation hall, which was also used for the public exams. On the Sunday night after the Retreat there was a film show and school really started the next day.

There were four full day classes until 4 pm and two half days Wednesday and Saturdays until 1 pm. There was study every night including a short study on Sunday.

Rugby

On the first Wednesday after the retreat the rugby season started. By this time all the new students were supplied with football kits, the cost being put on the bill to the parents. Then each student went individually to the lay brother, Peter, known as 'Brother Pete' who was in charge of the sports shop packed to the ceiling with all sorts of sports kits to be supplied with real football jerseys, shorts, stocking and boots. My trip to Pete's shop was the fulfilment of my dreams.

The management of the rugby was run on a club system, each club having at least thirty or more members. The first club was the prospective senior squad and trained and played on the best pitch and provided the prospective Cup Team. The second club was a lower standard, which could provide a seconds team. The third club was the prospective junior cup team and members had to be under a certain age. The fourth club was the under fourteens who played a limited amount of friendly matches. The fifth club was the under thirteens who played very few matches.

I was assigned to the under fourteens where some of us had to learn the rudiments of the game but I had seen many newspaper pictures of international games and frequently listened to radio commentaries so the change from Gaelic to Rugby was not very difficult.

All clubs togged out on Wednesdays and Saturdays and after a few weeks the senior and junior cup teams known, as S.C.T. and J.C.T. respectively would have friendly matches against other colleges almost every week. The under fourteens did not have

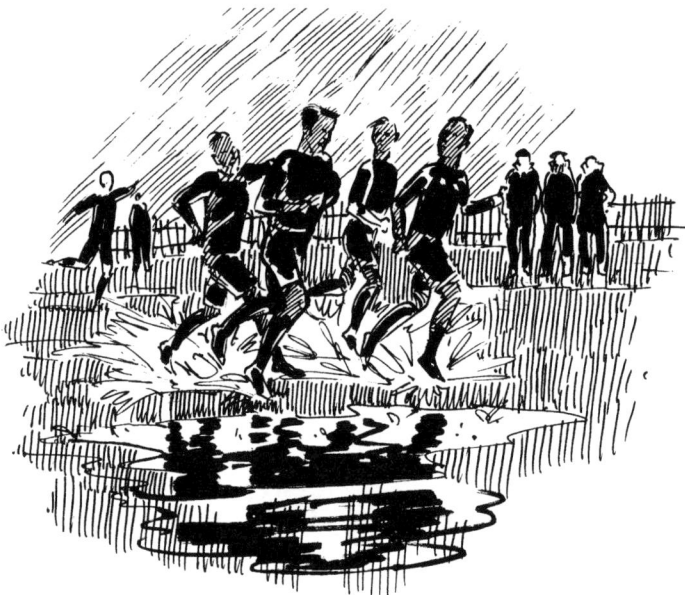

From Slyne Head to Malin Head, A Rural GP Remembers.

many matches but enough to keep up the enthusiasm to get on the team. I was delighted to get on the team for a few matches. It was a great thrill to get out with our trainer always one of the priests to play away matches. On those occasions we were back for the evening meal and late study. In the meantime, classes and study had settled in and I felt very happy and enthusiastic about the whole system.

I preferred the supervised study in a large study hall than to buckling down to study at home. The food was reasonable, good and varied and if I disliked a meal I just left it and made up for the loss at the next meal.

The war was still going on and the one effect that it had on the college was the scarcity of coal for running the central heating system so that the dormitories and classrooms had no heat. The only places to be heated were the college chapel and the study hall. As the weather got colder the one thing that I missed from home was the heat from the turf fire.

When Bernard and myself went out on our monthly day off, the routine was to travel on the bus into the city and meet Aunt Archie who would take us to a restaurant for lunch, usually Clery's, which she reckoned was the best place in town. Then on to a film of our choice, which invariably would be far from Archie's choice.

She would also come to visit us in the college once or twice a term on a Sunday, which was the official visiting day. After the first year we were able to get around the city ourselves and sacrificed the free lunch.

At the end of the first term there were two events, which took place annually, and these were first, the term house exams and the second the annual opera or more correctly operetta.

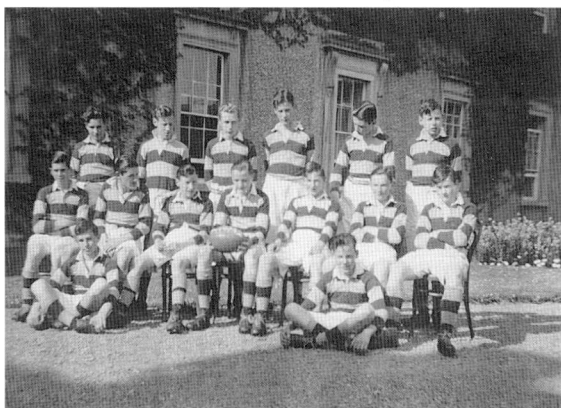

Junior Cup Team.(1943)

The written exams were a new experience, which I enjoyed and I was happy with the results when they were read out after the holidays.

'The Opera' was always a Gilbert and Sullivan operetta for which the students taking part were training and rehearsing for most of the term. It would be on for three shows and a dress rehearsal. The audience were invited parents and guests from around Dublin and a special night for the Sisters of Charity of St Vincent de Paul. Up to that time I had never heard of the G & S Operettas so this school production of 'The Gondoliers' instilled in me a great love for the G & S Musicals and every time I hear the music or singing extract from any of their shows it brings back memories of Castleknock and the Gondoliers production of December 1940. In the following years the Pirates of Penzance, The Mikado and the Yeomen of the Guard all brilliantly produced by our great history teacher the late Fr Donal Cregan.

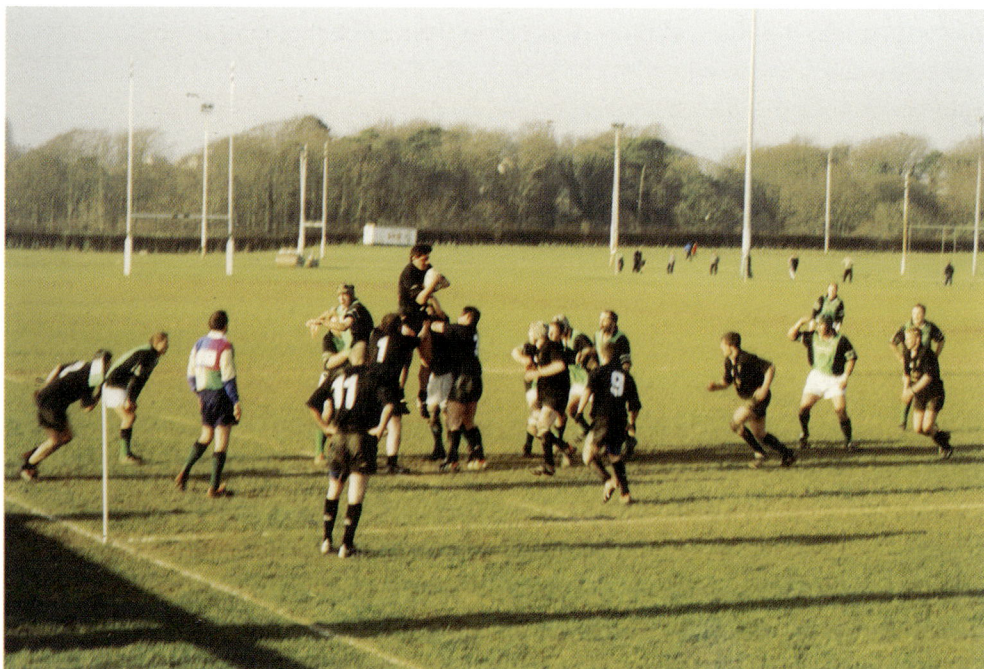

The Connemara Blacks vs City of Derry. (2003)

Next on the Agenda & Christmas Holidays

Next on the agenda were arrangements for going home. Due to the fuel scarcity all public transport was limited so for students from the north, south and west who travelled by train, the college had to make special arrangements with the railway companies for booking tickets for certain times and book taxis for transport from the college to the various stations. This entailed a very early start in darkness for everybody regardless of the times of departure of the various trains.

As the war was becoming a permanent fixture, the trains were gradually becoming slower due to lack of coal, so the journeys were becoming more tedious with slow travel and long delays at stations.

Heating on the trains became non-existent. The worst time of the year was returning from Christmas holidays, as the weather was much colder in mid-January.

I remember one year in particular, as far as I can recall it was 1942, it was snowing. We appeared to have been on the train for ages and eventually got on a taxi in Dublin to take us to the college as the roads through Phoenix Park were restricted the taxi driver tried to go via Chapelizod and stuck in the snow on the steep hill going up to the college but eventually got there.

In the early part of the war years, my father would meet us in Galway but when the cars were put off the road, we finished the journey on the bus and depending on the day we either got to Clifden and finished the journey by hackney to Ballyconneely, but if we were lucky to hit one of the two days that the bus came through Roundstone we arrived directly to our door.

On arriving home for the first time at Christmas the first great attraction was the blazing turf fire. The next change was a perception that everything around us appeared smaller due to the comparison with the long, wide corridors, wide stairs and large windows in the college.

Another notable thing was the drastic change in the landscape and this was not a perception. On looking out in the morning after arrival, the fields that were green and fresh when we left home were now almost black. The white washed walls were flaking and turning a green mould colour.

This change was perfectly normal for Connemara in those days due to the heavy rainfall and more severe frost than we are accustomed to in modern times.

After two days we were back into the normal routine and freedom of being at home but we were still happy with the boarding school system so that when the holidays ended returning to school was no problem.

We had the experience of one term behind us and now looked forward to the next term, which was going to provide a number of new experiences.

On returning the first thing we noticed was that the central heating was on so that the whole place was well aired and warm which was a great help in settling back into normal routine. After two days we returned to heat only in the chapel and study hall. This was just a minor inconvenience of the war.

January. Snow. Flu. and Starvo

January was frequently a month for snow, which usually arrived shortly after returning from Christmas holidays. This hampered the football and other activities but there was some compensation with snowball battles and when there was severe frost, skating on thick ice in a disused quarry on the edge of the college grounds.

January was also a month for Flu, which occurred on most years. The severity and duration of the epidemics varied. The infirmary, which was geared up for routine illness and minor flu epidemics, could cope for a while but if it was severe or prolonged junior dormitories, which were near the infirmary, were used. There was a full time nurse and an appointed G.P. who was available when required.

Severe widespread epidemics caused mayhem for a few weeks. I can remember having flu twice and at another time when there was no epidemic.

There was a brilliant system of catering in the infirmary, which appeared to work well. Every patient that arrived there was put on a diet of 'chicken tea' and bread for at least two days. The traditional name for this was 'Starvo'. It did no harm to the genuinely sick but concentrated the minds of the malingerers.

As January moved on the senior and junior cup squads got down to very serious training. The first stint before breakfast was a run around a wide walk known as the track. After breakfast there was a strenuous indoor session in the junior play hall.

This consisted of press-ups and various other exercises for building strength in legs, arms and backs, the session ended with a run outside up and down the hill outside the college twice, then in for a shower before starting class. The special training went on until the team or teams were knocked out of the cup. I did this training the one year I was in the junior squad and the three years in the senior squad 1942 – 1945. Out of the lot I played in one junior cup match which was against Newbridge in the first round of the cup in Donnybrook and lost 3 – 0. Not a brilliant rugby career by any stretch of the imagination but I enjoyed every minute of the training and being involved with the cup teams for four years. I felt that I was honoured to have played in many friendly matches over those four years.

Winning the Cup

While Castleknock usually had reasonably good teams and produced many international players in the early part of the last century, they have only won the senior cup on rare occasions. Usually they survived one or two rounds and occasionally reached a final. 1941 was one of those years when they reached a final against Blackrock who won it.

Bernard and myself felt we were very lucky to have this rare experience in our first year. The excitement mounts with each round until it becomes intense on the days leading to the final in Lansdowne Road, the oldest rugby ground in the world. For us the match reached the heights of excitement as we led by six points to nil at half time and the depths of anti-climax at full time as Blackrock won 9 – 6.

Three years later I was in the senior squad for the second year and had played in most friendly matches up to the first cup match and then lost my place. The team beat Clongowes in the semi-final to reach the final against Belvedere and win the cup. The enormity of the boundless excitement of that spring evening is beyond description but I have to attempt to describe the scenes of emotion that greeted the team as they were carried into the refectory with the cup was something else. The fact that I was within a whisker of being on it did not bother me at that time. The college had won the cup while I was there and part of the squad was to be a life long memory. I am now going to 'fast forward' my story by thirty two years to 1976.

In that year one of my sons, Ken Junior, was on a Castleknock team that reached the final against C.B.C Monkstown. I had hoped at that time that after thirty two years there could be a senior cup medal in the family, but it was not to be, Monkstown won by 3 – 0.

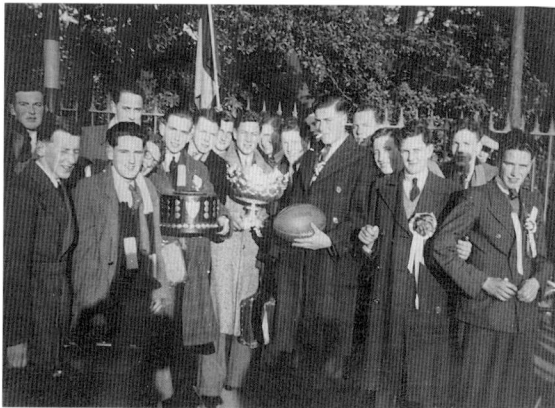

Winning the Cup. (1944)

Summer Term

Back to 1941 and coming into the summer term, there was a sudden change of scene. The rugby season is over and the high goalposts are gone. Tennis courts and athletic tracks are being laid. For those sitting the leaving and inter cert the moment of truth is drawing closer every day.

Bernard and myself had never played tennis so this was the time to learn at least the rudiments of the game. There was no official coaching so we gradually picked up the rules and some techniques from friends who had the skills. In a short time we could play the game at our own playing standard. Bernard was good at handball and enjoyed playing on the two fine alleys. He did very well in tournaments and reached quarter and semi-finals. I played more tennis but also went for athletics in the sprints and long jump and was on the junior athletic team in 1943 and on the senior team in 1945.

Night of Terror

On a Friday night at the 31st May in 1941, it was a Whit Weekend when the bombing of the North Strand in Dublin took place. During the night we were suddenly awakened by the sound of aircraft and of frequent explosions causing the large windows in the dormitory to rattle violently.

We were all terrified and were certain that Dublin was being bombed and that bombs were exploding very close to us. These explosions and the rattling windows appeared to be going on for a long time and then eventually gradually cleared. I am sure that it only lasted a short time but when you are convinced that bombs were exploding all around and you expect a direct hit at any moment so you had a perception that it was a long period.

I have not got the details of how many bombs were dropped or the number of aircraft involved but what gave us the impression of continuous bombing was actually explosions of anti-aircraft shells being fired at the bombers. There were a number of anti-aircraft guns situated in Phoenix Park and they would have been relatively near the college and probably close to McKee Barracks. On a later date, on a clear day, we saw and heard exploding shells. At another time and on another clear day we saw shells exploding near a highflying lone aircraft.

Bernard and myself had a day out on that Whit-Monday and went to see the devastation in the North Strand. Naturally, we could only view it from a distance but it was enough to give some idea what it was like for the residents in the area and for the relatives of those killed and injured. We had experienced this one small incident in the war, while in England, France and Germany bombs were raining down on towns and cities every night.

At the end of the summer term there were house exams at the same time as the public exams so that the term did not break up until the main parts of the leaving and inter cert. were finished.

Students doing the Matric Exam (long since abolished) remained on until it was finished but there were no rules or restrictions apart from returning to the college before a certain hour at night.

On the last evening of the school year before breaking up the annual prize-giving ceremony took place in the study hall when prizes were awarded for both academic and sports achievements.

The long summer holidays had now started. At that time everybody went home, as there was no such thing as working abroard for the summer due to the war. We returned home as usual by train and enjoyed the journey through the Midlands viewing the countryside in full bloom, at least until we passed Athlone. Usually at that stage clouds would appear coming up from the west and as we reached Oranmore the drizzle would start. Despite the weather conditions Connemara would still be beautiful having recovered from the long winter.

In Ballyconneely we were fully occupied at the turf in the bog, saving hay and frequently stints in the bar. In good weather we had swimming.

As Bernard was very keen to pursue a career in farming he left Castleknock after two years to go to an Agricultural College.

I continued on at Castleknock doing my best at studying and sport. I got out to every football final in Croke Park up to 1944 and saw Galway lose three finals in a row. Again due to the war there were no rugby or soccer internationals.

Athletics

I was on the junior athletic team in 1943 competing in the 220x4 relay and long jump without success. I had improved at tennis and enjoyed playing. Every summer I entered the competition to get more practice.

I was on the senior athletic team in 1945, my last year in the college. As regards the athletics this is the year I really remember. The Leinster Schools Senior Athletic Championships were held in the Guinness Iveagh grounds in Crumlin. These grounds had a modern Cinder Track, which in 1945 was considered state of the art. I was really excited and thrilled at the honour of competing on this track as I had only experienced running on grass tracks.

These championships were held on two Saturdays. The first day was for qualifying for the finals and we won our 220x4 relay heat easily in a time very close to the existing Irish record. We were really excited at this and practised our baton changing every day for the next week. Our coach was very keen on baton changing. On the final day we were really at the peak of fitness and full of confidence. As far as I can remember we were competing against Blackrock, Clongowes and Synge Street. I was the third runner and was level with an opponent on taking the baton and still level at the change over and it remained very close to the finish. We did break the record but unfortunately in second place so the winners set the record. We did get bronze medals and a great memory and that was the end of my career on the cinder track but not the end of running.

The Final Push

During that last year at school I studied extremely hard for the leaving. Latin was a compulsory subject for both Matric and Leaving. I could never get the hang of it as I was never a good listener in class.

During the last two years I literally taught myself with the aid of translations and learning off vocabularies and grammar books. I had never passed Latin in a house exam but I achieved a very good pass mark in the leaving and also passed the Matric. The President of the College was so amazed that he wrote me a personal letter of congratulations.

At the prize-giving ceremony on the last night of the last term of my fifth and last year in school my dreams of going to a boarding school had come and gone and had certainly lived up to my expectations. I also felt a deep sense of gratitude to my parents for providing the opportunity to avail of this experience.

My greatest moment at that ceremony was being presented with the one and only prize I had won over the five years and that was the bronze medal for second place in the relay race of the Leinster Schools Athletics Championships of 1945. Memories come back at where it all began, running races in Ballyconneely schoolyard. I got the leaving results in the week that the atomic bombs were dropped on Hiroshima and Nagasaki and brought World War 2 to an end.

What Next

Having got the Leaving and Matric, the next thing was to decide what to do. I had a notion for a while that I may have had a Religious Vocation but as St Augustine was reported to have said 'Not Yet O Lord'. It was then decided that I would go to university for a year to study arts. It was decided to go to Dublin because several cousins had been there and Archie was still around. I was delighted with the idea of going to U.C.D. mainly because it was the big centre for G.A.A. All-Ireland Finals and rugby and soccer internationals. At this stage I knew my way around the city centre and a sound knowledge of the way to Croke Park, Lansdowne Road and Dalymount Park.

Archie was instructed to obtain digs before the college opened, as I had no intention of going to any of the university halls of residence. While I enjoyed the boarding school and went by the rules for five years I did not wish to become institutionalised. Archie after much searching had come up with digs situated very near U.C.D. It was situated on Harcourt Road at the corner of Richmond Street. The front of the house was situated behind a large hoarding covered with all sorts of posters advertising the latest films in town, various cigarettes, gins, whiskeys etc.

To get to the front door of the house it was necessary to go through a door on the hoarding! A husband and wife ran the house. The boarders were three tradesmen and myself on full board. My room situated behind the hoarding was very small and cosy but the noise was terrific. Trams were still being used at that time so as they came screeching down Richmond Street and around the corner on to Harcourt Road with ear splitting clattering and banging and then a left hand turn on to Harcourt Street where the iron wheels resounded like they were shredding the tracks. Harcourt Street Railway station was also in the vicinity so the huffing and puffing and whistling of the trains frequently joined in the din.

U.C.D.

It was a very short walk from Harcourt road along Adelaide road to the college in Earlsfort Terrace. As I walked up the steps and into the main hall I was really excited and thrilled that I was about to become a university student. The formal admission and registering procedure in those days was very short and simple. Having stated the faculty of your choice and handed in your Matriculation Certificate and filled up a form you received a student's registration card and identity card.

I was now in a position to explore the building and peruse the profusion of posters inviting new students to join various sports clubs or college societies. My first priority was to join the rugby club with a view to playing on the Freshmen's Team.

This team was confined to first year students to bridge the gap between secondary school leavers and senior rugby. So I knew about this as they played against the senior school teams and other universities. I succeeded in getting on the team and trained once a week in the college grounds in Belfield with more senior players. We had a trip to Belfast to play the Queens Freshmen and had two matches against Trinity and several against school senior sides.

In first year I studied English, Irish, Logic, Modern Irish History and Latin with which I had no problem after two years of self-teaching for the leaving.

I have memories of Professor Dudley Edwards' lectures and teaching methods and especially his arguments and discussions with Brother F.X Martin who later became Professor of Mediaeval History. First Arts was not very strenuous as most of the subjects were a continuation and raising of leaving cert standard.

On the social side I joined the Literary and Historical Society, which was the oldest society in the college and founded in Joyce's time and always referred to as the L & H. It was a free show every Saturday night in the Physics Theatre. Well known politicians and other VIPs were invited as principal speakers and as with most universities large amounts of shouting and heckling were usually a feature. Such luminaries as Charlie Haughey, Garret Fitzgerald and Ulick O'Connor were students at that time and would have attended the L. & H.

Another weekend activity was the Friday night hop, or dance, in 86 St Stephens Green. This was the large period house in which the original university was founded by Cardinal Newman and where Joyce studied for his degree. There is a small bust of Joyce in the Green near the entrance gate opposite 86. Joyce was in U.C.D from 1898 to 1902.

In 1945 the main function was dancing, theatrical productions, a restaurant and reading room for the benefit of the students. In recent years this building has been completely refurbished and is called Newman House. A small church designed like a miniature basilica and known as University Church is situated near Newman House and religious ceremonies associated with the college were held there. While U.C.D had magnificent space in Belfield for playing fields and recreation which many years later would become a huge Campus it had the use of the public park of St Stephen's Green which was just a few yards away from the college and frequented by many U.C.D and College of Surgeons Students.

At the end of my first term in college I had no doubt that I was going to enjoy my time in university the same as I had in boarding school. By now Bernard had finished agricultural college and was working at home and concentrating on the farming and tolerating the pub.

Christmas in Connemara

At this stage we were attending the big dances in Clifden Town Hall. At first our parents were still dancing but gradually had given up. For a few years the big event at Christmas was a Fancy Dress Ball, which we all attended. We always had a 'half-way house' in our cousin's house in Clifden, which had been our mother's original home, and we always called there on our way to the big dances. There were two girls and two younger boys. The two girls had been boarding in the convent school in Kylemore Abbey run by the Benedictine nuns. As recent or past pupils they were invited by the nuns to attend the (real) Christmas Midnight Mass in the Abbey, they could take two guests, needless to say Bernard and myself were the two guests.

It was certainly a unique experience in those days in Connemara to drive the twenty miles to Kylemore, seeing all the houses lit up with candles in every window and driving into this 'fairy tale' castle and Abbey lit up for Christmas in a forest at the foot of a mountain which is renowned on picture postcards all over the world.

Change of Abode

On returning to Dublin after the Christmas holidays and arriving late I returned to my digs behind the billboard to be informed by the landlady that she had rented my room to another client. She had decided that she could not hold vacant rooms during student holiday times. This was a bit of a shock at around 9pm on a cold January night. Fortunately I could have gone to Archie's who was now living in Rathmines which was not very far away but I decided not to bother her at that time of night so I went to one of the many small hotels in nearby Harcourt Street hoping to search for digs the following day.

There were two evening papers in Dublin at that time; 'The Evening Herald' (still there) and the 'Evening Mail' (long since gone). The Mail had the most ads for accommodation so I started scanning the mail the next day and tried several places without success. I then decided to inflict myself on Archie and after nearly a week I succeeded in my search and found a place very near my original abode and had a wonderful time there for the next two years.

32 Synge Street and Shaw

This was a unique house, which was situated beside the house where George Bernard Shaw was born, and the name of the street honouring another Irish playwright John Millington Synge. A landlady and her sister-in-law ran the house.

There were some medical students and a law student in residence and I was looking forward to having company. The day I took up residence I developed the worst 'flu' I ever had. There were three beds in the room on the first floor but the other two were not occupied. Being in a strange house and not having met the other occupants and with a high temperature after about two or three days I became delirious. The landlady then got very worried and decided to call the local G.P who assured her that I had just a bad flu and not a terminal pneumonia. When I got on my feet I got two friends who had been at Castleknock and were pre-medical students to occupy the two vacant beds so then the house had its full compliment of five medical, one law and one arts students.

This was a two-storey house with a basement and a front 'area'. There was a large kitchen in the basement, a range and a gas cooker. There was a small garden at the back of the house. Partially in front of the house there was a large over ground air-raid shelter. It was a long concrete rectangular building, which was waiting to be demolished.

We all had meals in the kitchen with the landlady and her sister-in-law, there was always great conversation with fun and banter at these meals and we enjoyed meal times.

At a later date there was an incident that I will never forget. It occurred on a Sunday morning at a relaxed breakfast. The landlady had become weary (or said she had) of the bad language being used by all the boarders, that it was a disgrace for so called educated people to be using this kind of language in her presence etc. etc. While the expounding was in full flight one of us lit up a cigarette butt (which was a common practice during rationing) and after inhaling a prolonged drag on the butt and by now with the small butt held between his fingers swung out his arm to rest his hand which landed on the back of his neighbour's hand with the red hot butt lodging itself between the victim's fingers who jumped up from the table roaring every expletive in the book and calling the smoker by every derogatory name and expletive imaginable. In the meantime there was an explosive roar of laughter all around the table. The sister-in-law was in hysterics and I was also in hysterics and had to lie on the floor to relieve the pain in my ribs. The landlady sat gob-smacked and when the din died down she shook her head and laughed and said 'what's the bloody use in talking to you lot'.
We all enjoyed the laugh, there were no hard feelings and we all lived happily for the

remainder of the academic year. I was enjoying my social obligations of attending the L & H, the hops in 86, going to the occasional film and enjoying the rugby on the Fresher's team while not neglecting the lectures and slogging stints in the Arts library. During the summer term as the going got tough I loved walking in the green in May when the wallflowers and tulips were in full bloom while the relaxation helped to calm the exam butterflies. I passed the exam and that was another milestone having put a university exam behind me.

Pillion Journey to Limerick

After the exams of the summer term a school friend who was also in U.C.D studying engineering had got a second hand army motorbike and he suggested that we would both go on the bike to Limerick to visit another school friend who was then training in the Shannon Catering School. As these bikes were clapped out and would not be capable of much speed so in trepidation I agreed to go.

As usual in June the weather was bad, it was cold with heavy showers. I certainly had no leathers but fortunately I did have at least what I thought was a heavy overcoat but was still totally inadequate for the unseasonable weather conditions. After a few instructions on how to balance the bike on corners we set off heading south to the plains and The Curragh of Kildare. Despite the meagre shelter behind the driver I felt the cold wind and the rain rapidly soaking into my overcoat. Although better clad, my companion also felt the cold wind and the rain so we made numerous stops on the way to get the circulation going in our nearly paralysed limbs.

We called to another school friend in Castledermot who supplied much needed hot tea. Unfortunately this was the only acquaintance we could call on on the long journey and Limerick was still a long way off. On this journey I vowed many times to myself 'never again'.

We reached Limerick sooner than expected and then headed for Shannon to meet our friend somewhere around the kitchen of the fledgling airport. Probably as a result of the bouncing on the pillion seat all day my brain appeared to have got blurred for recalling events of that evening except for a vague memory of going to a dance in a very packed hall in Limerick and later in a friend's flat either in a bed or on the floor. The return journey was completely different, the weather had changed back to real summer conditions so the trip was very pleasant but it was to be the end of my first and last pillion ride on a motorbike.

Summer Holidays 46

On returning home I got into the usual summer work on the bog and the hay etc but with the addition of a new recreation which was a pleasant surprise. There had been a tradition of a tennis club in Clifden, which had lapsed for some years and was now about to be revived. So Bernard and myself were invited to join the revived club. The system was that every Thursday, which was the business half day in the town the club held a 'round robin tournament' in the afternoon, weather and work permitting. We cycled five and a half miles to Clifden when possible. We were delighted with this and enjoyed gaining more experience of the game. The tournaments went on for the whole summer afternoons and frequently until nightfall. On some occasions the club ran short dances or hops in the town hall to raise funds. I have no idea how long this revival lasted but as far as I could remember I enjoyed it for three to four years.

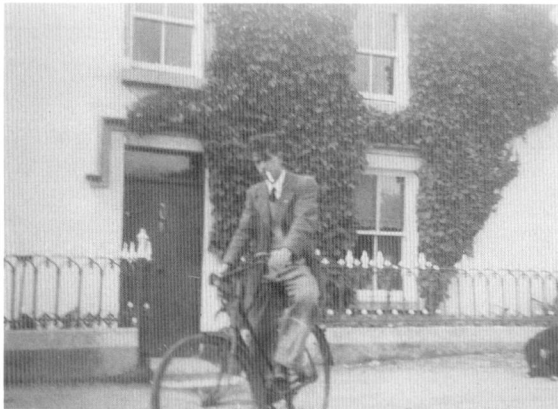

Ken's House, Ballyconneely, Galway.(1945)

Deaths in the Family

During the forties and early fifties there were a number of deaths in the family, all on my mother's side. Her brother Michael, a GP in Newport, Co Mayo, died suddenly in 1944. In July '46 her sister-in-law, May, her brother-in-law, Joe Casey in 1948 and her brother James in 1950. There was a death every two years and they all occurred in the summer months. Her sister Rita Muldoon died in February 1953.

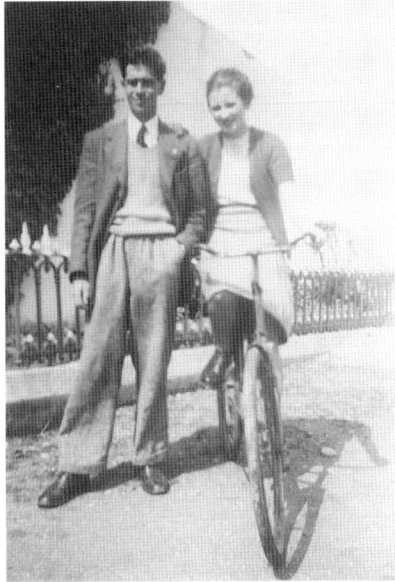

Ken's and Cousin Marie.(1940's)

Climbing 'The Reek'

This famous mountain of pilgrimage also called Croagh Patrick where according to tradition St Patrick fasted and prayed on its summit. It is roughly forty miles from Clifden so that it was traditional for many people in Connemara to go on pilgrimage and climb to the summit on the last Sunday in July. I always had a desire to do this pilgrimage but I admit it was more for the adventure rather than for the religion.

In July 1946 Cousin Nolly Lee, also called Nora, a short time after her mother's death asked me if I would accompany her to do Croagh Patrick. I jumped at the idea and said I would be delighted. At that time the pilgrimage was on a Saturday night on the eve of the last Sunday in July so that climbing took place in semi-darkness from around 10 or 11pm. Nolly's plan was that I would sleep in her family home on the night before departure and that we could take our bicycles on a service bus from Clifden to Leananne and then cycle the twenty nine miles from there to Newport where we would stay for the weekend or longer with our aunt-in-law Sarah and her two sons and do the pilgrimage from there.

In the morning everything went according to plan and on reaching Leananne we got our bikes and headed north to the end of the Killary at Aasleagh. The weather was reasonable, it was not raining but we had the inevitable showers which were not too frequent so it was pleasant to be cycling towards our destination along the Westport Road and really enjoying the mountain air and the scent of the heather. We demolished our sandwiches and milk during a bright interval sitting on a large flat rock on the roadside. Sometime after resuming our journey we began to feel tired.

Eventually when the peak of Croagh Patrick suddenly appeared it came as a shock to contemplate that after miles more cycling we would have to climb to this peak in the dusk. As we went on pedalling, the peak appeared to be getting higher.

Eventually we arrived in Westport and pressed on to the last nine miles to Newport to be resuscitated by the welcoming Aunt Sarah. The final plan was that we would travel by car with Cousin Patsy to Murrisk where the climb starts around 10pm. I had very little sleep the night before so I had very fitful sleep in the car to Murrisk. When the car stopped I woke up to hear people shuffling and talking all around us, carrying heavy walking sticks and many had flash lamps. It was pouring rain and I felt very cold. I could hear people selling sticks and shouting 'shticks for the reek', 'shticks for the reek', 'shticks for the reek'. For a few moments I had no idea where I was and when the reality began to dawn on me I was hoping it was all a nightmare from which I would soon wake up which I did very quickly and found myself in the real world in Murrisk and about to climb a mountain in the pouring rain.

I cannot recall if we had shticks or not but we moved on with the crowd and began to enjoy the experience. At first the climb was gradual and it led on to a right hand turn along a relatively level ridge which brought us to the real climb up to the peak and this

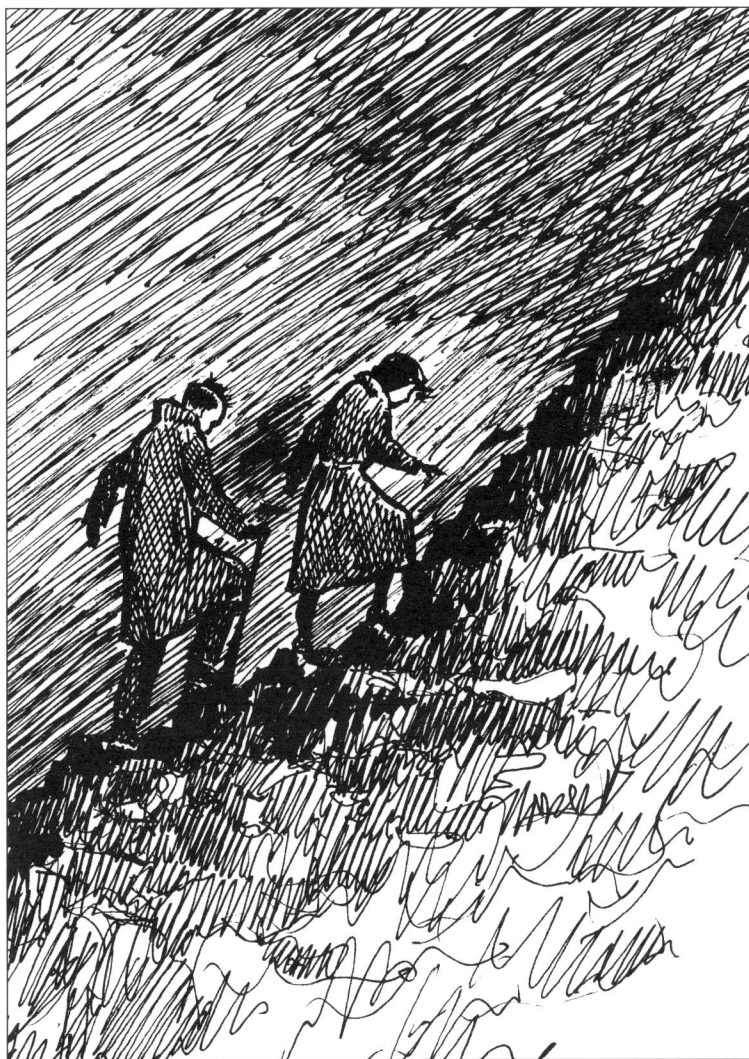

entailed half walking and half crawling and stumbling up a mass of coarse shale and stones until finally reaching the summit.

It was still dark and there was a thick mist, which made it difficult to see the small church, or oratory where the pilgrims walked around several times reciting prayers. On arrival we were warm after the exertion of the climb but soon felt the chill of the wind and the bog. I am certain that St Patrick had plenty of sheepskins to wear when he was fasting up there.

We were young and fit and there for adventure including a few prayers and a new experience and we certainly learned a lot from seeing so many elderly people, men and women, who do this every year and large numbers of pilgrims did the climb in bare feet after walking long distances. I either read or was informed that at one time pilgrims coming from a long distance visited Ballintubber Abbey on their way to the Reek and left there footwear there until their return from the pilgrimage.

As dawn began to penetrate the cloud we descended the mountain hoping to get a view of Clew Bay and its numerous islands but that is a very rare sight, as it appears to be part of the penance to be denied this wonderful view. We got safely back to Sarah's and after a large breakfast, slept until teatime. I did the climb again on each of the following two years going on a special bus from Clifden direct to Murrisk. On my third and last trip I was rewarded with a brilliant view of Clew Bay. Like everything else, climbing the reek has become easier as the climb must now take place in daylight to reduce the number of accidents that occurred at night.

My mountaineering was not yet finished as around forty years later I climbed Muckish in Co Donegal and Yeats' beloved mountain, Ben Bulben, in Sligo. I can still get to mountaintops but only by cable car.

U Turn

The summer of 1946 was now moving on and I had to decide on a definite course for a future career. I had never contemplated becoming a doctor despite the fact my family were saturated with doctors for three generations. My mother had two uncles and two brothers and my father had one brother. I had six cousins, all older than me.

For good measure I also have vet and dentist cousins. For some reason I had a fear of hospitals and doctors, which may have been due to Bernard's recurring illness, when he was young. My whole outlook changed during the first year in First Arts, probably because of my association with so many medical students in the digs and rugby club. Having successfully completed a year in university I had a huge amount of confidence to study medicine. During the summer holidays I was also encouraged by some of my doctor cousins. Before the end of the holidays I had made a definite decision. With this change of outlook and sudden development of confidence I felt like the apostles when the Holy Ghost landed.

The College of Science

I returned to college and 32 Synge Street in October to renew acquaintances with the landlady and to be welcomed into the medical student fraternity by the other students. In those days changing to another faculty was a minor formality. The change from school subjects to scientific subjects required some mental adjustments but that was easily overcome by the new interest in the practical side of the scientific subjects.

At that time most of the premedical lectures and laboratories were carried out in what was at one time called 'The Royal College of Science'. This building is the major part of what is now, government buildings which face onto Merrion Street and Merrion Square and with its big blue dome is now seen daily on TV bulletins. That is where the UCD premedical engineering and other science students walked in every day, through those big gates and up the steps to enter what was then the College of Science. While there was no CAO or points required to get into medicine in those days there was no guarantee that we would get out at the other end or worse still get as far as first medicine. There was usually around three hundred students taken in to pre-med but the exam at the end of the year was competitive. The first hundred got through in the June exam and twenty in September.

When one looked up at the full lecture theatre and realised that only a third would get through in June it certainly concentrated the mind. This is where I felt that the experience and confidence gained the previous year would be a tremendous help.

As I was no longer eligible for the 'Freshers' rugby team I rejoined the main club and I became a regular on the third A's team. This was the lowest possible grade in the club but I was very happy about that. We trained every Wednesday and played a match every Saturday and as there was no pressure we all enjoyed our games.

1946 – 1947
The Royal and the Capital

I was still interested in following GAA, soccer and also had an interest in the rowing club, as I knew some of its prominent members. I usually went to the Wiley Cup Universities Championships in Islandbridge to encourage UCD. During 1946-1947 the rugby and soccer internationals were returning and I remember going to my first soccer international which was the first post war match and was against Spain and played in Dalymount Park, known to the Dubliners as the 'Dailer'. The Irish captain was the legendary Jackie Carey. There was a huge crowd at this match and I remember there was a big crush going in and we just got in before the gates were closed and were broken down a short time later but fortunately nobody was injured.

The first post war rugby international was probably in early 1947 before the snow. As you can imagine life was not all sport. Study was always a priority and I was taking the science subjects very seriously attending all lectures and studying in the college of science during the day and in the Arts Library at night. Pre-meds did not use the special medical library until first medical. The subjects were physics, chemistry, botany and zoology.

My pastimes were not all confined to sport. I also went to films and the theatre with one of the Synge Street students, Charlie Sullivan. We went to plays in the Abbey and the Gate. On returning from the Christmas holidays Charlie and myself did a tour of the pantomimes in the Olympia and the Gaiety. Jimmy O'Dea was still going strong in the early days and assisted by Maureen Potter. Needless to remark we were patrons of the dizzy heights of 'The Gods' where the admission was one shilling each for the seat on a hard bench. During the opera season in April and May we always went to one 'La Traviata' in the Olympia.

There were two theatres come cinemas where there was a combination of a stage show and a film and was fantastic value having two shows every day except Sunday. They were The Theatre Royal usually called the Royal and the Capital. The Royal situated in or near Hawkins Street near O'Connell Bridge and off Burgh Quay. The Capital was situated in Princess Street beside the GPO. The Royal was a very large building with a huge seating capacity and promoted many first class shows. The usual format for introducing the standard show was a large theatre organ played by Norman Metcalf, which gradually ascended from the pit to introduce the famous dancing girls, the Royalettes. The much-loved Dublin comedian, Noel Purcell, was featured frequently.

There was also another outstanding annual promotion and that was the world famous Joe Loss and his orchestra with their signature tune In the Mood. I never missed going to this show, there was another feature at the royal, which had a long run. If there ever was a forerunner of the modern, Who Wants To Be A Millionaire, this was it.

The show was Double or Nothing and was compered by Eddie Byrne, who later became an actor and played in several films.

This was a quiz show where the compere invited people from the audience to go up on the stage and answer general knowledge questions to win money, which the competitor could keep or opt for another question to double or loose all. Students anxious to earn some money by placing their general knowledge (or lack of it) on the line supported this show very well. It was a well-known fact that Eddie disliked students by taunting the competitors with derogatory remarks and wisecracks.

My memories of the Capital were of the main artists Sean Mooney who sang the Millers Daughter for ages, Cecil Sheridan, a brilliant comedian who always appeared wearing a huge cap with a peak two to three feet long. When he stomped out on the stage as John Joe Mahoky he always brought howls of laughter from the audience. Harry Bailey was another comedian who went for risqué jokes. Joe Bonny was a brilliant drummer and his big act at the end of a drumming session was to drum his way around the stage using the drumsticks on any props that came into view and eventually finished up by drumming across the floor and back up to his seat at the drums. Another great artist in his own right was Mickser Reid, a small man, who played in many comic sketches.

The foregone description of students' social life in Dublin (in the rare aul times) is not intended to indicate that I was doing nothing else.

Study and attending lectures was always my first priority, I rarely studied in the digs but used the college libraries, which had the added benefit of a walk to and from the library.

The Glimmer Man

This period was when domestic gas was rationed during the war and for a considerable time afterwards. Coal was also rationed and the available turf was so wet it was almost impossible to light and then gave little or no heat. Gas was mainly used for cooking so when it was rationed it was only allowed on at mealtimes and for a short period. The supplies were controlled by the corporation but when turned off small quantities filtered through the cookers and this meagre supply was referred to as the glimmer and could be used to boil a kettle if it was left on long enough.

This practice of using the glimmer was strictly forbidden so the corporation sent around inspectors known as 'The Glimmer Men' to regularly check up on customers that could be breaking the rules. If caught at this practice the gas would be cut off completely for a period of punishment. The fuel rationing in Dublin at that time caused severe hardship from the cold, as there was no such thing as insulation. I am certain that our landlady would have used the glimmer but I am not certain if she was caught. I knew for sure that the house was like every other house, very cold and was about to get much colder.

The Snows of '47

This snowstorm was probably the worst in Ireland in the twentieth century. While there would have been many snowstorms lasting a week or two, this one lasted for almost eight weeks. As far as I can remember it started on the 24th January and continued almost unabated until it ended in a blizzard on St Patrick's Day. I was fortunate to be in the pre-med class that year because The College of Science was very well heated probably because its central heating system was on the same circuit as the Dail in Leinster House. We could use the library there during the day but it was closed at night. The Arts Library in Earlsfort Terrace was open but was too cold. Coal was already rationed and as the coal mines in England became completely frozen up due to the subzero temperatures and as the available turf was almost useless, there was no hope of studying in the digs so after the evening meal the only place of refuge was the cinema where there was a reasonable amount of heat, probably generated by the audience.

Most of us (all non-drinkers) went to the pictures almost every night and twice on Sundays. When we had seen all the films in the city we moved out to the suburbs and coming near the end we were seeing the same films for the second time. In those days each cinema had separate films not like modern times where one film would be in several cinemas. On Sundays we went to a matinee in the afternoon, which was always chaos and mayhem with screaming children running over and under the seats. I kept a diary at that time and in those eight weeks I saw forty-two films. I did not return to a cinema for two years.

On Sunday mornings we all purchased the Sunday papers, which were very small in those days due to scarcity of paper. We brought them all back to the digs and rolled them up tightly to make a small fire in the living room to keep us surviving until lunchtime. During that freeze-up there was snow on the footpaths at all times and when it was fresh it soaked in through shoes and even got into galoshes which were fashionable at that time. I remember that there were some very bright clear sunny days with subzero temperatures but without snow.

These freak days appeared to occur on Saturdays which was invariably followed by a blizzard on Saturday night so as we woke up on Sunday morning, daylight was partially blacked out by the amount of snow adhering to the windows and on opening a door the snow came tumbling in.

At that time there was no big parade on St Patrick's Day, it was a closed day for pubs, the one well-known exception being a bar at the annual dog show in the RDS in Ballsbridge. I have no doubt that the show organisers were delighted with the increased funds. The main event of the day was the railway cup, hurling and football provincial finals in Croke Park, which were postponed due to the snow. It was customary for the cinemas to open in the morning on St Patrick's Day so on this morning of the holiday Charlie and myself went to a film in the Metropole and had a snack after the film. Later we proceeded to the afternoon show in the Royal. A short time after the show started that part of the city was blacked out by a power failure due to thunderstorms and a blizzard that heralded the end of the snows of 47.

Easter

The Easter holidays soon followed so I was certainly glad to get home to see a real turf fire and really get stuck into study in a big way to catch up on lost time. When I got back to Dublin after the holidays there was still heaps of dirty frozen snow on shaded footpaths and the Dublin Mountains were still covered with snow.

Fortunately I caught up with the studies and the exam and would move on to first medical to become a real medical student.

The First Flat

On returning to 32 Synge Street in October the group in the digs broke up due to some of them going into residency in hospitals. Two of us, Charlie and myself joined two other med-students and moved into a flat in Ranelagh. This was very unusual at that time as very few women and almost no men students lived in flats. None of us were good cooks but we never starved. The flat was in 2 Woodstock Gardens, Ranelagh and within walking distance of UCD. We had morning and evening meals in the flat and a meagre lunch in the restaurant in 86. On Sundays we had a feast of steaks, potatoes (spuds) and mash turnips for lunch. The kitchen was very small and we actually shared it with two bus conductors who came and went at completely different times and had most of their meals in canteens. Charlie and the two other students were from Co Tyrone. The occupants changed on a few occasions.

The Connemara Blacks

There were a number of male college students from Clifden who had been in rugby playing schools chiefly St Joseph's College, Garbally Park, Ballinasloe, Black Rock College, Dublin, Castleknock and Clongowes. Probably around December 47 or January 48 some of these students decided on forming a rugby club in Clifden and organised a number of experienced players and some keen newcomers in GAA ranks and organised a match against Westport Rugby Club.

Much to our delight Bernard and myself were invited to join the scratch team to play Westport. The club was to be called the Connemara Blacks.

The original 'Connermara Blacks' was and is a black and red fishing fly used on the lakes and rivers of Connemara. We played that first historic match on what was once the Clifden racecourse and now a holiday home complex, called Clifden Glen. I remember the ground was soft and there were several pools of water around but that did not deter the players who were making rugby history. As far as I can remember we did not have a return match during the same holidays but we certainly had one the following year when we travelled to Westport on a bitterly cold day with hail showers. The following year we travelled to Ballinasloe on a day of frequent snow showers to take part in a seven-a-side tournament. I presume we had two teams, that was to be my first and last time playing seven-a-side rugby, which required a higher level of fitness than we had to keep running around what, appeared to be a huge ground. The formation of the Connemara blacks was reported in some English papers at the time. After those early few years I lost touch with the actual club but I continued to follow their fortunes in the newspapers.

They progressed to become an officially established junior club in Connaught rugby. In recent times they reached the final of their grade but did not succeed. However, they were more successful in the year 2001 in winning their way to the All-Ireland League. I have very happy memories of Bernard and myself playing a very small part in the founding of the 'Connemara Blacks'.

On 29th April 2002 they won the top four of the All-Ireland third division of the All-Ireland League in Lansdowne Road and on 11th May 2003 they won the Connaught Senior Cup when they defeated the Buccaneers Rugby Club for the championship.

The Triple Crown

When the Rugby Internationals returned after the war Ireland appeared to be doing well with a great young team, which included the legendary out-half Jackie Kyle, then a young medical student in 'Queen's'. Also included was another medical student in the College of Surgeons, Carl Mullen, a brilliant Hooker and Captain of the Irish team for a few years.

For the benefit of the uninitiated the Triple Crown was a mythical honour given to the team that defeated the other three international teams in Britain and Ireland. Ireland had not won this honour for fifty years. In early January 1948 when reading the fixture list of Rugby Internationals for the coming season, I noticed that Ireland and Wales would meet in Ireland's last match of the season in Ravenhill, Belfast. I also saw an ad in the paper that there would be a special train from Amien Street (now Connolly) to Belfast for this match and the cost of the excursion would be one-pound return. This was during the Christmas holidays so I put one pound aside until this date towards the end of March.

Ireland beat, England and Scotland and so my dream came true of winning the Triple Crown we were now heading for the Grand Slam against Wales.

To add to the occasion it was the start of the Easter holidays so I released my pound on the big day to join Charlie and the throngs in Amien Street Station and it was all-aboard for Belfast and Ravenhill. After a close and dour match with the score at 3-3 well into the second half, the big forward J.C. Daly got the ball in a line-out near the Welsh line and crashed his way over to score and left it 6-3 for Ireland until the final whistle and the Grand Slam for Ireland.

There was an almighty roar as crowds swarmed over the pitch while J.C. Daly was carried aloft to the tunnel. I finished up on one of the crossbars with an unknown man holding a tricolour between the two posts. This was to be Ireland's most historic Rugby victory in the old order. It was to be won again 26 years later in Lansdowne road in 1974. I was not at that match due to pressure of work and inability to obtain tickets. I did have the facility of T.V. I was happy in the knowledge that I would never see the like of 1948 again.

After the final whistle I had lost Charlie. He was going home to Tyrone so I followed the crowd to the station for the return rowdy journey back to Dublin and the Easter holidays. Rugby has moved with times and has developed in various directions with professional players world cups etc. One could say it is still Rugby but a 'different ball game'.

Horses and Races

My father was not a gambler by any stretch of the imagination but he enjoyed a moderate bet on horses and for a number of years never missed the Galway Races and during the war years in the forties brought Bernard and myself which during those years was a unique experience.

When petrol was rationed we travelled by bus and stayed in Galway for two or three nights for the duration of the races. During those days the city took on a massive carnival mood, which was boosted by the huge number of sidecars (Jaunting Cars), which were used for transporting thousands of holiday race goers from the city to the famed Ballybrit Racecourse, which was made more famous in 1979 when the Pope himself addressed the multitudes there. The sidecars appeared to be owned by people

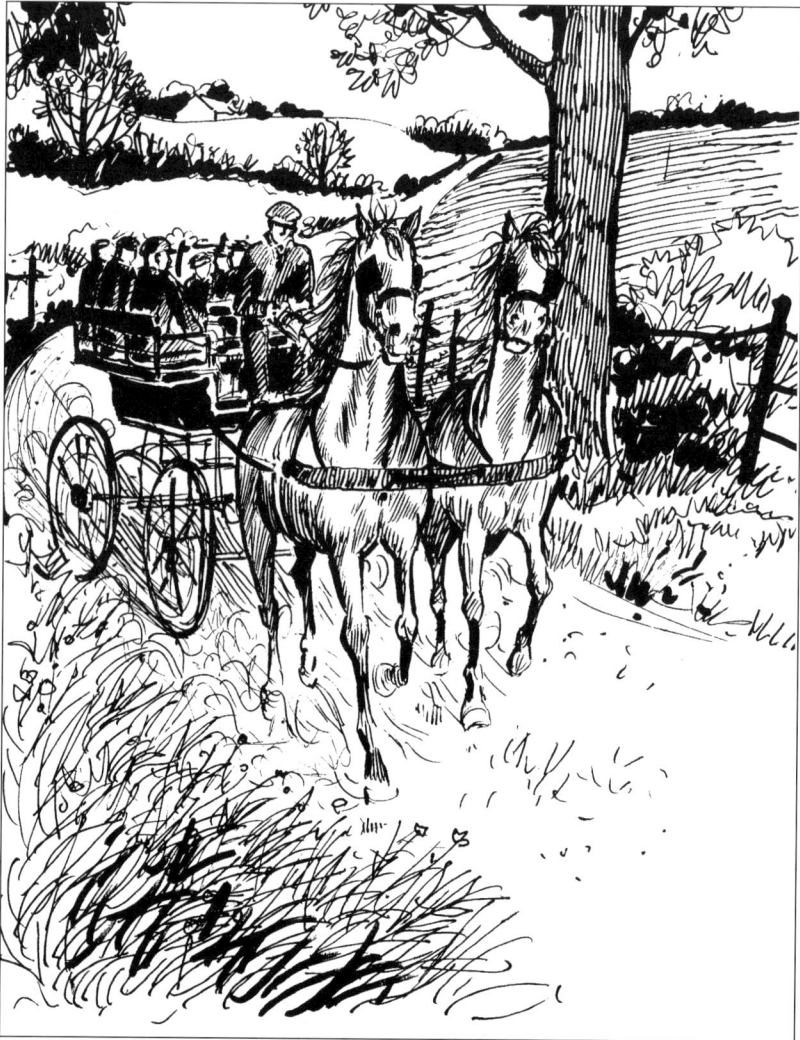

From Slyne Head to Malin Head, A Rural GP Remembers.

from around the Galway area who were awaiting a brilliant opportunity to boost their incomes. From early morning they were gathered in large number all around Eyre Square as the owners and prospective passengers usually bargained about the fare similar to the Killarney Jarvies.

The journey to Ballybrit could vary from a pleasant jaunt to a hair-raising nightmare depending on the speed and your ability to hold on. It was certainly more exciting than sitting in a small car in a two-mile tail back and the first race about to start and no mobile phones to place a bet with your friendly bookie. After the races the nightlife, which plagued Bishop Michael Browne, went on all night with dance halls and ballrooms going on until the early hours.

A race week feature was the huge marquee inside Eyre Square. The sidecars plied their trade for most of the night between Eyre Square and Salthill.

There was also another race meeting that we attended and that was Ballinrobe, Co Mayo. This meeting was held twice yearly, the first usually during the Easter holidays and the second in early July. These meetings were in complete contrast to Galway. The venue was much smaller and more relaxed and so was the sixty mile journey along the Twelve Bens and then along by Lough Corrib to Ballinrobe. In July 1951 we got a brief view of the filming of 'The Quiet Man' in the Maam Valley.

Olympic Games

As my memories go back to the 1932 Olympics and the feats of Pat O'Callaghan I have since then taken an interest in this great event. In 1948 it was great to have the games return after the twelve-year break due to war. The venue was London and at that time would have been a very small event compared to the Sydney games of 2000 but with fifty-nine nations and around four and a half thousand athletes taking part it appeared large. Ireland did not win any medals but would have had a big increase in competitors compared to 1936.

My two big interests in this Olympics were 1) rowing and 2) the feats of Holland's great Olympic athlete Fanny Blankers Cohen known as 'Flying Fanny' who won four gold medals, the 100 metres, 200 metres, 80 metres hurdles and the 4x100 metres relay. I had the great privilege of seeing her running on grass in Lansdowne Road at one of Billy Moton's Athletic Promotions.

My interest in rowing in the London Games was the fact that Ireland was to be represented in one event of the rowing by whoever won the Irish senior Eight's of 1948 and that year it was won by UCD. I had a personal acquaintance with two members of the team and with the manager. All three were medical students. In those days rowing was confined to the universities and a small number of clubs. Since then there has been a huge change in the sport and has advanced to challenge for gold medals in most categories.

HELSINKI 1952 would be remembered by the feats of the Czech, Emil Zadapek winning the 5,000 and 10,000 metres.

MELBOURNE 1956 – 'Can we ever forget?' I remember setting the alarm clock for 4.05am to hear BBC Radio commentary of the 1500 metres in which Ireland's great hope, Ronnie Delaney, was competing. With the ear splitting, cracking and tearing I could just make out the commentator's excitement at the finish as Ronnie Delaney came down the last straight to win the 1500 gold medal. That was a brilliant Olympics for Ireland as our boxers did us proud in winning two bronze medals and one silver medal. I remember the New Zealander Peter Snell winning the 800 metres and 1500 metres.

MEXICO 1968 – watching live on TV, seeing Bob Beamon's great leap of 29ft (5 metres) to set up a New World and Olympic record which lasted for many years.

MUNICH 1972 – this should have been a famous Olympics for athletes but it was marred by the Munich Massacre when eleven Israeli Athletes with their Arab captors died in a shoot out. The games were stopped for a few days of mourning and then continued on. The outstanding athletes were Mark Spitz of the USA winning seven swimming gold medals and four world records. Olga Karbut, the Russian gymnastic, came to fame.

The Bearded Flying Finn, Lasse Viren, won the 5000 and 10,000 metres. Mary Peters, the English lady from Northern Ireland and loved by everyone from north and south won the gold for the toughest event of all – The Pentathlon.

MONTREAL 1976 – All Ireland had great hopes of Eamon Coughlan winning the gold medal for the 1500 metres in Montreal. He was our leading athlete for several years and had a brilliant career at indoor running in the USA. In the 1500 metres final he had the misfortune to get 'boxed in' in the last few hundred metres and finished fourth. He appeared to be destined not to win an Olympic medal but he did have one day of glory at the World Athletic Championships in Helsinki in August 1983 when he won the World 5000 metres title. I remember the day very well as I watched his victory on the big TV screen in Croke Park, from behind the Canal goal, as my two native counties, Galway and Donegal, were on the pitch playing in the All-Ireland Semi-Final. Galway won but lost the final to Dublin in what was to be one of the dirtiest finals ever played. Donegal's day was yet to come.

MOSCOW 1980 – This was the year of the two famous English middle distance runners Steve Ovett and Sebastian Coe in the 1500 metres and 5000 metres. They were two great athletes and there was intense rivalry between them.

LOS ANGELES 1984 – After 52 years the Olympics returned to Los Angeles and again an Irish Athlete was to the fore in the City of the Angels when John Tracey did us proud by winning the Silver Medal when he finished second in the marathon.

I followed the whole race live on TV in the early hours and I can see John entering the stadium in second place and running to the finish to the huge ovation from the stands. While ringing in my ears was what must be Jimmy McGhee's finest hour as he recorded the feats of the past Irish athletes which must have gone back to Finn Mc Cool.

SEOUL 1988 – We all had great hopes of John going one better and taking the gold in Seoul but it was not to be. I have my own memories of this marathon. It was on a weekend while I was attending the Donegal Clinical Society educational weekend in Dungloe, Donegal. During that weekend I was suffering from shingles.

Fortunately there was a TV in the hotel bedroom and the shingles were ensuring that I would not fall asleep. John was not in good form either and was out of the race at an early stage.

Despite that disappointment he had a great record winning two worlds cross-country championship medals with his Olympic silver medal.

STRIKING GOLD
BARCELONA 1992 – This was another good year for Ireland as two of our boxers won medals. Michael Carruth won the gold medal by defeating a Cuban in the final of his weight. Wayne McCullough won silver in his weight. This was the year Sonia O'Sullivan made her Olympic debut and was very unfortunate to miss a bronze medal in the 1500 as she got boxed in to fourth place at the finish. Despite this set back she had a long career ahead.

ATLANTA 1996 – This was a very unusual Olympics for Ireland. We never made an impression at swimming but in Atlanta Michelle de Bruin Smith won three gold medals and one bronze which was a huge haul of medals for Ireland particularly for swimming. This was expected to be a great Olympics for Sonia but she became ill at the start but despite this she competed and qualified for the semi-finals of the 1500 metres but could not finish the race. After Atlanta she took a year off and had her baby Ciara and then went on to win the 5000 and 10000 metres in the European championships.

SYDNEY 2000 – The Sydney games have been acclaimed as the most spectacular and efficiently run games to date. Sonia had put all her problems behind her and was back in top form for her third Olympics and she was honoured to carry the flag into the stadium at the opening ceremony. Despite not winning a gold medal she did break the hoodoos of her previous two Olympics and ran two magnificent finals in the 5000 and 10000 metres winning a silver medal in the former, missing the gold by the narrowest of margins. In the 10000 metres she finished sixth to set up a new Irish record. She is now at the peak of her career and expecting another baby and I am now looking forward to the next games in Athens where the first Olympic Games of the modern era were held in 1896. I have my own personal Olympic triumph when in 1960 with my wife Eileen we walked in and around the ancient stadium in Olympia and examined the pedestal on which the Olympic torch is lit by the sun's rays at the start of each Olympiad.

The Real Medical Student

On entering first medical in October 1948 I was now a real medical student as the main subjects were anatomy and physiology. To study how the human body worked and make or break time was on entering the anatomy department in Earlsfort Terrace and inhaling the pungent smell of the formaldehyde used to preserve the bodies of the dead subject. The next shock was on entering the dissecting room to begin the long haul of the one and a half years of the combined first and second medical year's studies. The study of anatomy was to learn all about bones, joints, arteries, veins and nerves as well as the various organs. Trained demonstrators and technicians gave teaching instruction. Physiology was about how the body functions and the parts played by different organs. Also included was embryology, which was the development of the human body from conception to a newborn baby. Having passed the second Medical in March 1949, I was now considered a senior medical student so the next move was to attend a hospital to be introduced to clinical tuition and for the first time examine a patient.

The big decision was now to decide on which hospital to choose. Dublin students would appear to be spoiled for choice, as there were nine general and three maternity hospitals, three paediatric, one fever and one orthopaedic. The general hospitals were St Vincent's near Earlsfort Terrace and Stephen's Green, The Mater near Dorset Street and opposite Mountjoy Jail, Mercers and the Adelaide near the Gaiety Theatre and College of Surgeons, Dr Steven's beside Kingsbridge Station (now Heuston), Sir Patrick's Dunn's off Merrion Square and Mount Street, The Richmond off the North Quays, Jervis Street between Abbey Street and Mary Street which would be the nearest hospital to the city centre. The Meath off Camden Street and the hospital with the greatest history as many of the medical staff gave their names to medical discoveries like James Dixon Hypothyroid, Stokes Adams Syndrome, Collis Fracture, Chene Stokes Breathing. The Old Coombe in the Liberties, Holles St in Merrion Square, the Rotunda in Parnell Square at the end of O'Connell Street, the paediatric hospitals were Temple Street, Harcourt Street, and Our Lady's Hospital Crumlin.

It was generally accepted that students from each of the three medical schools, Trinity, College of Surgeons and U.C.D went to hospitals where most of their professors were consultants. I had been strongly advised by my medical cousins to follow this tradition and choose either The Mater or St Vincent's but having lived in digs and flat with students senior to me who had gone to Jervis Street and hearing about life there and the huge practical experience that could be obtained there due to the smaller number of students. I also heard about the friendly relationship with the consultants. I was very impressed by all of this and had almost decided that I would prefer to be a big fish in a small pond rather than a small fish in a big pond.

The summer term following the second Med-exam was very relaxed with introductory lectures in the important disciplines of medicine, surgery and obstetrics and we were free to attend any of the hospitals for limited tuition before making a final decision. St Vincent's Hospital being situated beside Earlsfort Terrace was a very popular choice for many students.

It was a well known hospital and had a great medical tradition of brilliant consultants but I ruled it out because of its structure of a number of small houses and a very small casualty department where there could be no real 'action' and excitement like the ambulances tearing down Abbey Street with sirens screaming and then in the big gate and screeching to a halt outside the famous Jervis Street Casualty Department.

The Mater was a magnificent modern hospital with a large casualty department but the only criticism I could make was the huge number of students around the beds and the Consultant, which made me feel a very small fish in a big pond.

The Richmond was a large and very old hospital and made up of different buildings. The numbers of students were a reasonable size and it was also more difficult to reach. Despite this I attended a few clinics there as well as a few in the Adelaide. At the end of my biased investigation of the pros and cons of the available hospitals it was Jervis Street for me or as any self-respecting Dublin man would call it 'The Jervo'. Despite being an old hospital it was a fine, very tall building with a brilliant view of the Dublin Mountains from the top wards and also a view across the roof of Independent House of Nelson while he was still on top of the Pillar.

Due to the rapidly moving times of the second half of the 20th century the old hospitals were having difficulty coping with modern technology so it was decided to amalgamate the Richmond and Jervis Street into one hospital in Beaumont. The vacant Jervis Street site is a massive shopping centre but fortunately the facade of the original building has been retained.

By coincidence I was frequently in Dublin while the building was in progress so at each visit I went down Abbey Street to have a nostalgic look at the old facade and almost hear the ambulances again screeching to a halt outside the casualty department or see myself pedalling up Mary Street on my bicycle to a clinic.

Jervis Street was originally founded in 1718 and called 'The Charitable Infirmary' and after moving to a few different locations finally settled in Jervis Street situated in the Mary Street, Capel Street and Abbey Street areas. In 1742 George Handel gave the first public performance of his immortal Messiah in Fishamble Street Music Hall to raise funds for Jervis Street and Mercers hospitals.

During that summer term 1949 I was really enjoying the thrill of attending the various hospitals and particularly Jervis Street where with a few fellow students we frequently visited the casualty department to see the action and even attended a few post-mortem examinations. We also toured around the wards and got basic tuition from the Registrars.

This homeliness was the beauty of Jervis Street. I had frequently considered joining the athletic club as I had missed the athletics after leaving school. There was always too much study to be done in the summer terms so to keep my priorities right I never joined but in this 1949 summer term I played some tennis in Belfield and went to some of the Sunday night hops in the old house in Belfield.

I also went to occasional hops in The Four Courts, which was a strange place to be partying, but there was a hall or a room around the back, which was used by law students who usually invited some medical colleagues to attend.

I have a vague memory of going for a swim with my friend Aiden Meade in the 'Forty Foot' near The Joyce Tower in Sandycove.

This was the place where only men were allowed to swim. We naively thought that we could enjoy a swim there but we experienced a near thing to drowning when we belly flopped into the freezing water and before recovering from the shock we were being swept out on a big wave and fortunately swept back to the rocks on another wave where we immediately scrambled out on to dry land. After this experience I could well understand why Joyce in the Tower scene of Ulysses described the 'Snot Green Sea' as the scrotum tightening sea!

After the relaxation of a summer holiday in Ballyconneely working on the bog, saving hay, the odd fishing trips in a curragh for mackerel on Mannin Bay, tennis in Clifden, several stints of filling pints and times changing cattle from one field to another and dipping sheep etc. I was looking forward to returning to college in October to start into third medical year and the clinical teaching in the hospitals. In third med the subjects were pathology, which was the study of how various diseases affected the body and its organs. This involved considerable time studying with a microscope.

Pharmacology was the study of the few drugs that were available and learning off a certain number of prescriptions for cough bottles, stomach bottles and others for nervous complaints. This subject has long since moved into a different world or planet and is a hugely complicated subject with multi-million pharmaceutical companies and corporations all over the world playing a very large part in the Irish Economy. Therapeutics was the study of how to treat various diseases and conditions.

Senior Student

On returning to the hospitals in October the student would have made their various decisions about their choice of hospital. The accepted large majority between the Mater and St Vincent's an average of 50 for each hospital. 'The Renegades' as I always referred to the small groups who went our separate ways were thirteen to the Richmond and seven to Jervis St.

I was back to the flat in Ranelagh. I was now 'mechanised' with a bicycle for cycling to the clinics in Jervis St every morning to be there at 9 am. It was a straight course on the bike down Ranelagh Road, Charlemont Street, Camden Street, South Great George's Street then on to Dame Street and a sharp turn to the left and down Parliament St. on to the Quays across the Ha'Penny Bridge on to Capel St Bridge then up Mary St and into Jervis St to wait inside the main hall to join up with the housemen and resident students or to wait for the Consultant. At that time the Medical Consultants were Dr. Billy O'Dwyer, Dr. Tommy Ryan, and Dr. Bob Davitt a descendant of Michael Davitt of the Land League.

The Surgeons were Mr. Des Murray, Mr. Dan Ryan and Mr Arthur Chance, the orthopaedic surgeon. Karl Mullan, who was Captain of the Irish Team and Kevin Quinn a famous centre were housemen. Both Davitt and O'Dwyer were very keen rugby fans so around the international season there would be brief rugby discussions before clinics on a Monday morning after an international.

In addition to the UCD group there would be a few students from the College of Surgeons and in those days, students from UCG did part of their training in Richmond and Jervis St. The numbers attending the clinics would still be small so that we were having personal attention.

Mr. J. C. Flood

Around 1948 to '49 we heard frequent stories from our senior students about a legendary surgeon Mr. J.C. Flood who had been a surgeon in Jervis St some time previously. According to the stories he was an English man who had come to Dublin after the 1914-18 war to study medicine and law. He studied in UCD and obtained an MCH (Master of Surgery) an MD (Doctor of Medicine) and also became a Barrister. Eventually, some time in the thirties he was appointed a General Surgeon to Jervis St and during that time he had built up a reputation among students of his opinion on various topics (true or false) particularly about his attitude towards women and Jesuits. The students of that time embellished many of the stories so that they became legendary. I had heard many of these from a senior student long before I went to Jervis St. In the early forties he up and left Jervis St and went off to enter the Benedictines in Downside Abbey in England but after a short time he returned to Dublin and recommenced surgery in Jervis St. During this time he had a part-time appointment as a demonstrator in Practical Physiology and during that time while in either first or second med I remember distinctly seeing and hearing this legendary man. We students were working at some experiments with microscopes and writing notes on whatever while Mr. Flood was inspecting the work he noticed a particular student (not I) who had very poor handwriting and he asked him where he was educated and the student replied Belvedere and Mr. Flood replied 'I could not expect anything better from the Jesuits'. He made no remark to me as he probably thought I was a new Picasso. After a short time he re-entered the Benedictines.

We all went our separate ways and I often wondered if he was still in the Benedictines until 1978 I read a newspaper report of his death. This report stated that he was ordained in Rome in 1951 and that Dom Peter Flood OSB BA MD MCH JCC Barrister at Law died on 16th December 1978.

This was a great and exciting time for the students as we felt that we were by now soaking up the knowledge as it was then. It was also a very busy time. When the clinic was over we would frequently practice our stethoscope skills on a few patients who were in those days delighted to have students examining them. We usually arrived at the hospital by different routes but returned to Earlsfort Terrace in a bunch up Abbey St. to O'Connell St. and the bridge down to Westmoreland St. then College Green, Nassua St, Dawson St and the Green to Earlsfort Terrace.

There were numerous small side clinics to be attended on certain days like Paediatrics in Harcourt St. or Temple St. Children's Hospital and in Clonskeagh Fever Hospital. Psychiatrics in Grangegorman as it was then called. This was a difficult trip on the bike going from one side of the city to the other. I have memories of some of the teaching Clinicians like Eric Doyle, a brilliant young Registrar, in Harcourt St.,

Professor Jack Henry from Trinity who lectured on Paediatric Surgery. Bob Colles a Consultant Paediatrician and former rugby international who came from the family of Abraham Colles who first described The Colles Fracture. I have a special memory of John Dunne the chain smoking chief Psychiatrist who gave up the 'fags' every Lent

1949 to 50 Back to the Butterfly Days

The summer term of 1949 was the one-year in which I could relax and enjoy the Green in a calm state of mind. The 1949 holidays came and went so it was back to College time in October and into serious lectures of Pathology, Pharmacology and the major subjects of Medicine, Surgery and Obstetrics and continuing the hospital clinics. I was still in the flat and studied in the medical library in Earlsfort Terrace, which was a pleasant walk from Ranelagh on to the Appian Way, Leeson Park and Leeson St.

In May 1950 the butterflies returned with the third medical exam which was passed successfully. The great thing about medical exams was the prompt release of the results, which could be on the evening of the last exam or at least within a few days. I was now looking forward to going into residency in Jervis St. in October 1950 and hoping for a long hot summer but forgot the old adage of 'The Best Laid Plans of Mice and Men'.

The Summer of 1950 and Death in the Family

There was a spell of very fine weather towards the end of June so Bernard and myself decided that we would get all the hay saved while the weather lasted and then get the turf out of the bog as soon as possible. All went well for a few days but then the weather broke and it rained for the rest of the summer and on into September (the next worst summer that I can remember was in 1985.)

We spent most of the 1950 summer twisting, turning, and the shaking of .wet hay in all directions in vain attempts to get it dry. The turf was in worse condition and never dried properly and by September the bog was so wet that even the donkeys were unable to do their usual work to carry it out to the roadside. The only alternative and the last resort were for ourselves and a few men to do the 'donkey' work and hump it out on our backs.

As usual in mid August we attended the Connemara Pony Show, which was traditionally the highlight of the season in Clifden. As usual for this summer of 1950 the day was drizzly and dreary. We were in and out of our Uncle James Lee's house frequently during the day and had arranged going to the big show dance in the hall with our cousins. In the evening we went home to have a meal and change for the big dance. Shortly after arriving there was a phone call from our cousins to tell us that their father had died suddenly.

James Lee was our mother's brother and we almost lived in that house and called there every time we were in Clifden so we were all devastated particularly as his wife May had died a few years previously. His death brought about a huge change but then that's life.

After that miserable summer I was looking forward to going back to college in October and particularly going into Jervis Street as a resident student. In those days students did their six-month residency after passing third med. having attended clinics for over a year I was certain that I was going to enjoy it. There was a small matter of an exam in March '51. The subjects in this were basic forensic medicine and public health medicine.

T.B. and the Student

On taking up residency in Jervis Street I was delighted to be playing a very minor part in the life of the hospital. Students and housemen were accommodated in dormitories. Registrars had private rooms. There was a common dining-room and sitting room. The housemen's dormitory was on the first floor and students between third and forth floor and in an odd situation with a very low ceiling. It was known to generations of students and housemen as 'Fagen's Den'. It eventually became historic when it was converted into the new Nephrology Department in 1963, which would become involved in the first kidney transplant in Ireland.

Each student was assigned to a consultant and his or her duty was to accompany the consultant, his registrars and housemen on his or her daily round. The other tasks were to accompany the housemen when admitting new patients. Another task was taking blood samples. When I found myself assigned to Dr. Billy O'Dwyer I knew I had hit the 'Jackpot'. He was a brilliant teacher of Clinical Medicine who could get across the basic skills and knowledge to students and junior doctors. At that time in the forties and fifties T.B. was rampant in Ireland and was fast reaching epidemic proportions until Dr. Noel Brown got himself elected to the government of the day and took the T.B. problem by the 'scruff of the neck' by having many new Sanatoria built and organising country wide mass x-rays.

At that time UCD had established a health bureau in the college, which was situated in 86 (Newman House) and managed by a consultant Physician from the Mater Hospital, Dr. Michael Moriarity fondly referred to by the students as 'Mike'. If a student did not feel well he or she consulted Mike and he would advise them what to do.

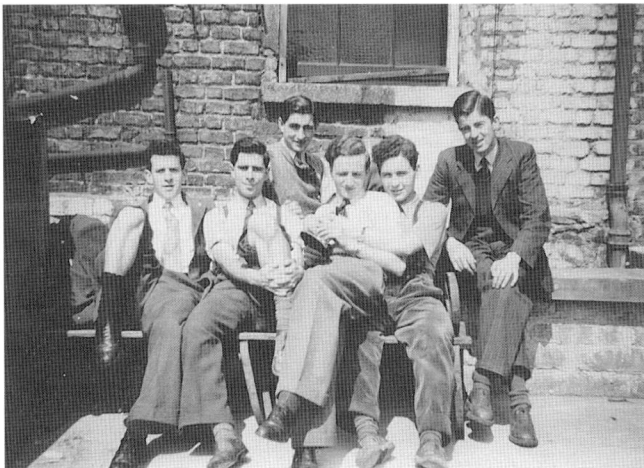

Aide Meade. Ken O'Flaherty, Vincent Meagher, Tony Farelly,
Tomo O'Brien, Ciaren Barry, Medical Students. (1950)

From Slyne Head to Malin Head, A Rural GP Remembers.

During my first three months in Jervis Street I became conscious of some loss of energy, which I thought was caused by the central heating. One night in December another student who had been called to a ward noticed that I was sweating profusely and awakened me to enquire if I was feeling all right and suggested that I should have a chest x-ray and that he would get one as well. Within a few days we had consulted Mike who gave us x-ray request forms to take to the Mater and to call back for the results in a few days. My colleague's x-ray was clear but mine showed a shadow which in medical terms was a T.B. Infiltration or (Shadow). This was a very early stage of the disease, which would clear up on rest Mike reassured me but told me to take the x-ray films to Dr O'Dwyer and that he would look after me, which he did. Blood and Sputum tests were normal so the only treatment required was complete rest at home.

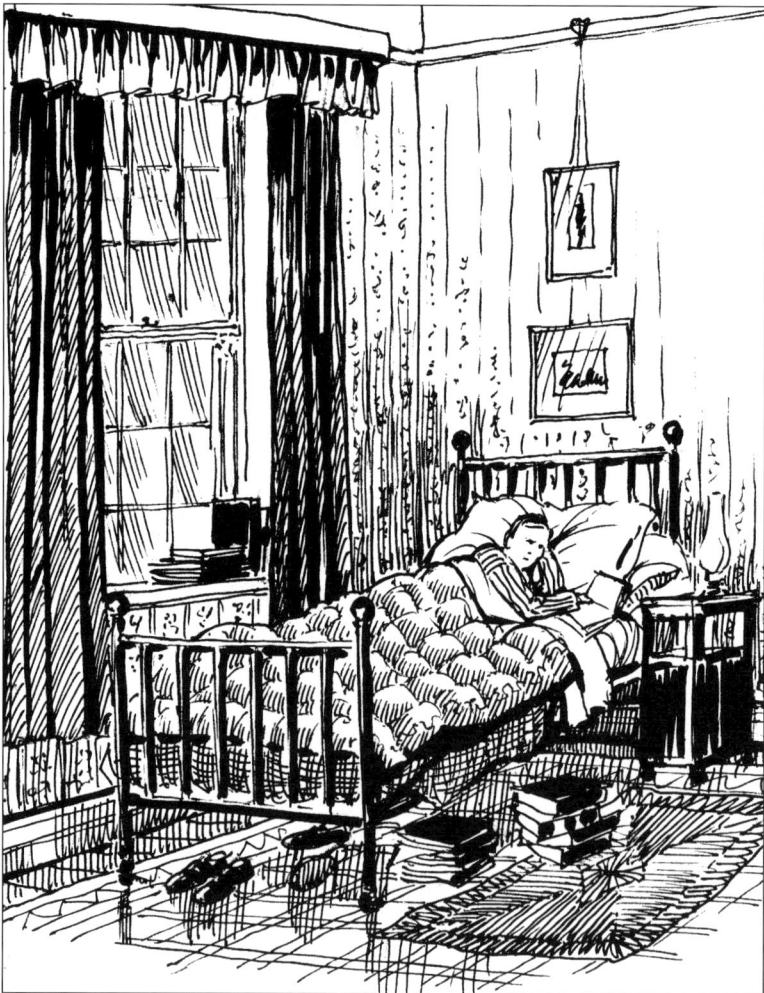

While the result of the x-ray was a bit of a shock and would be an upset, interrupting my training I was relieved that the disease was diagnosed at an early stage and was certain to heal. Fortunately I had finished three months of the residency which was the compulsory length required so that the second three months could be missed. This was the one easy year in the medical course with an exam in March 1951 on basic Forensic Medicine and Public Health. So it would be possible to do enough study at home and return in March to succeed in the exam and have a check up, this was arranged with permission from the dean of the faculty. Dr O Dwyer advised me to take plenty of rest but not necessary to stay in bed.

I reckoned that if there was one prefect time in the year for staying in bed December and January was it so I stayed in bed from before Christmas until February reading the books on public health and forensic medicine then gradually resuming normal activity and returning to Dublin in mid-March to succeed in the exam and have a check-up which showed that the lung was now almost clear.

I was now back on schedule and due to enter the Old Coombe for obstetrical training for three months. The reason for choosing the Coombe was the big fish in the small pond principle. I ruled out the world famous Rotunda because of its large size and I did not consider Holles Street because all training there was in hospital with no real practical experience of home deliveries that was necessary for training at that time.

As I write I would be completely against home deliveries. Holles Street has been immortalised by Joyce in Ulysses when Bloom pays a visit to the student's hospital residence, he is annoyed by the 'shenanigans' of the students.

Students at Large 1951

On entering the Coombe, the students were given a short introduction and training in the labour wards before going out in pairs on bicycles to the deliveries on the district which covered a large area from York Street near Stephen's Green all the Liberties, Inchicore, Crumlin, Ballyfermot which was still under construction and Kilmainham. The rule was that each student had to attend twenty complete deliveries in three months and write a record of each case.

There was a back-up system in the hospital consisting of four or more experienced doctors known as Clinical Clerks with two always on call in the hospital to deal with any emergencies on the district. They were provided with a small ambulance, which was actually, a van fitted with two stretcher beds.

The rest of the equipment consisted of a large, metal box containing several obstetric instruments the whole lot were sterilised and the lid sealed with adhesive tape. In addition there was a supply of drip sets and transfusion fluids and ether for open anaesthesia. This was carried out by dropping the ether from a bottle on to a mask which consisted of a piece of lint stretched over a metal frame. When using ether an open fire had to be quenched as the ether could cause an explosion. At that time I considered that the most important equipment for the student was at least two pennies or more to phone the hospital for help in an emergency. Despite the lack of sleep and the general stress of the training I enjoyed obtaining such a huge amount of practical experience.

The types of houses and accommodation varied according to the district where the patient and family resided. It could be a broken down tenement, one roomed flat on the third or fourth floor somewhere in the Liberties with no light on the rickety stairs or a brand new house in Kylemore Road in the Ballyfermot Estate. This estate was in its early stage of development. Kimmage and Crumlin were well established so most of the houses were very comfortable. One of the worst buildings was Keogh Square in Inchicore. It had been an old Army Barracks converted into flats and at that time was about to be condemned.

There was one very remarkable feature about the maternity facility in most of the tenements and that was the 'Labour' room, which came as a pleasant surprise after climbing the long creaking stairs. We entered the room and frequently found it newly painted or wallpapered with an electric ring, or even a fire, for supplying warm water, laundered towels, fresh bars of soap and to crown it all a Handywoman would be in attendance. She was usually an elderly lady who in her day would have had a large family.

She would give us the obstetric history, as she knew it, of the lady in labour and very frequently give lurid details of past obstetric complications either about the women being attended or about a near disaster of a close relative. Most handywomen were very helpful and gave assistance and in addition addressed us as 'Doctors'. When there was a prolonged labour she would reassure us that 'she does be very tedious doctor'.

Bicycles were our mode of transport. As regards finding our way to the tenements and estates we were either given very good directions or a neighbour or husband cycled to the Coombe and then accompanied us on the outward journey.

The 'on call' for the students was on a rotation system which could be very irregular because when a pair returned to the hospital after completing a delivery and then writing details into a log book, the next call could be immediately or a long time depending on how many other students were called out while we were away so that on some occasions we could be next 'on call'. That possibility was the real training for the single-handed G.P. of those days. In addition to the practical work there were lectures and demonstrations going on in the hospital given by the Master or Assistant Master.

The Final Push

Having completed the Coombe training at the end of June I was now into the final year and determined to get stuck into the last great push. On returning home I started into serious study, which was to go on almost relentlessly for a full year until June 52.

During the summer months I had certain times for taking short walks and a few very short social breaks, going to one or two big dances. On going into residence in Jervis Street I had left Woodstock Gardens and planned to return to digs for the final year. On returning to College in October I got digs in Mornington Road, Ranelagh, which by coincidence was just a few, yards away from Woodstock Gardens. There were three of us, Charlie Kehoe who was a Jervis Street student, also my partner in the Coombe. The third was my cousin James Lee who was starting Veterinary and was in pre-med in UCD.

In this final year I was still attending clinics and lectures in the various hospitals and studying at every spare moment during the day, except for the short time after lunch in 86 that I took the 'butterflies' for a stroll on St Stephen's Green and a draught of the scent from the wallflowers. At night we studied in the digs and went for short walks around the block to revive our drooping spirits. The three of us had two things going for us we all had a sense of humour and were non-drinkers. Coming close to the final I was becoming stressed with loss of appetite and energy but just kept going.

In those days the Final Med went on for three weeks so it was really exhausting. All went well for me up to the last day of the exam in Stephen's Hospital I had an altercation with a surgeon examiner that sent me back to the 'drawing board' to repeat this subject six months later in November. I should have been shattered but I felt that in my state of health I would have to take that length of time off in any event. I was due a check up for the T.B. with Billy O'Dwyer and the x-ray confirmed that it had flared up slightly so he advised six months rest.

I returned to Ballyconneely once more but I did not stay in bed this time and I took plenty of rest. This was one of the rare, long, dry summers.

I got up late every morning and had a slow walk through heather, furze and numerous wild flowers to a sheltered area and read novels every day and did not look at a medical book until I returned to Dublin in October three weeks before the repeat exam. I took up temporary residence in Mornington Road and did leisurely study until the exam, which I passed.

I had another x-ray, check up with Dr Billy O'Dwyer and he found that the T.B. lesion had healed up very well but to be on the safe side he advised me take another six months off as in his opinion the stress of going into a hospital house job could cause another break down.

He then reassured me that when I returned in July 53 I would be his houseman for six months. I was conferred on the 19th of December 1952 and returned to Ballyconneely for the last time from UCD.

The long haul of seven years from the billboard in Harcourt Road to the conferring photograph on the steps of Earlsfort Terrace has left me with many happy memories.

Doctors at Large

I now felt very well and was anxious to start work as a doctor so the time appeared to drag on very slowly but at least I learned to drive a car and drive a tractor, which gave my morale a boost. I helped Bernard on occasions and returned to social activities which had almost ground to a halt between the T.B. and the escalation of study as the Final Med approached. July eventually arrived so it was back to Dublin for another x-ray now showing that the lesion had almost vanished so the time had come to start work in Jervis Street as a Houseman.

During that year between repeating the exam and the extra six months I had lost touch with most of my classmates who by July 1953 had gone their separate ways. I had never lost touch with Charlie Sullivan or Aiden Meade. Charlie had returned to the north and had got a G.P. job in the N.H.S. in Strabane, Co Tyrone as an assistant. Aiden was still in Dublin and working as a Houseman in Monkstown Hospital near Dun Laoghaire and he had asked me to do two weeks locum for him before I started in Jervis Street.

This was a real baptism of fire but I survived it and was relieved to get going in Jervis Street under the watchful eye of Dr Billy O'Dwyer.

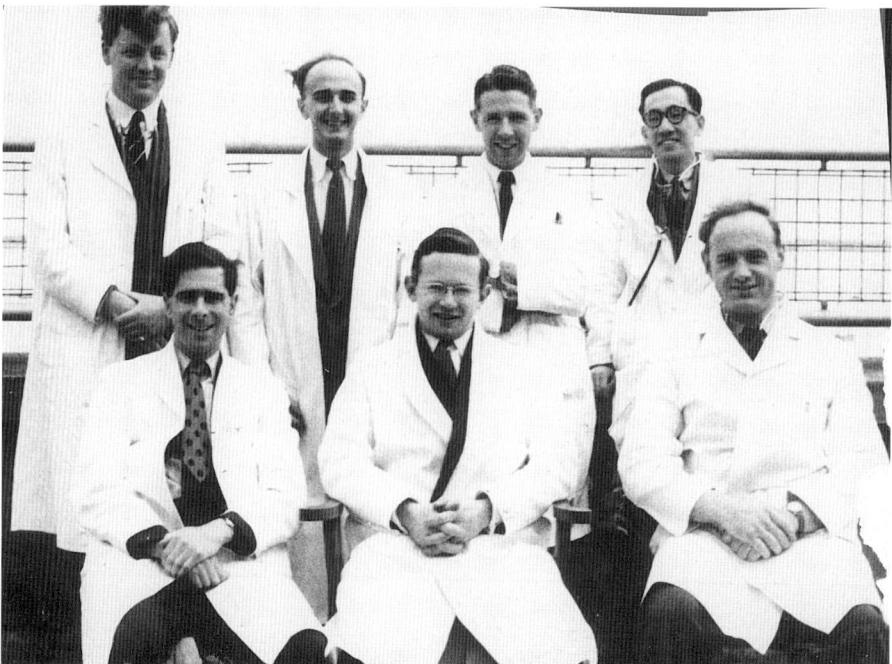

Ken (bottom left). Junior Days at St.Michael's Hospital, Dunleary

Hospital Doctor

It is now difficult to imagine in the 21st century that up to the fifties there was virtually no drug available for direct treatment for high blood pressure. One did appear while I was in Jervis Street so that physicians were carrying out surveys on its efficacy.

This drug known as Vegalysen was produced by May and Baker one of the few companies around and had produced Sulphonamides in the thirties. Dr O'Dwyer was carrying out a survey. For several days I was commissioned to check a woman's blood pressure every hour with the patient in three different postures, lying down, sitting and standing. This had to be recorded several times daily in order to see if the drug was too strong or too weak or if it was tolerated by the patient. These types of surveys would have been carried out in hospitals in several countries. It was proved not to be very satisfactory so it was withdrawn but it was a start and now fifty years later scientists are still working to get the perfect drug for many different conditions.

Another chore for the Houseman was examining every patient on admission and discussing the findings with your student, taking blood from veins and giving intravenous injections, mostly for heart failure and asthma. Oral antibiotics had not yet arrived but penicillin had arrived in injection form and fortunately Streptomycin by injection had or was about to arrive and played a very large part in treating severe pneumonia, T.B. and bronchitis and went on to improve its benefits when numerous other antibiotics arrived.

During that six months I was learning something everyday and becoming more expert at communicating with the patients and coming near the end of the six months I preferred the medical side to the surgical side and contemplated eventually specialising in general medicine.

At the end of the six months term Housemen either changed to another speciality in their own hospital or left to apply for a job in another hospital. I had decided that while I was very keen on minor surgery I had no intention of ever doing major surgery so I decided to leave and apply for another medical job, which I got in St Michael's Hospital in Dun Laoghaire. I had no regrets. I loved every day that I had working with Dr Billy O'Dwyer.

Doctor in Love

In July 1953 before I went to Jervis Street I was out with Aiden Meade and his girl friend Maura. He had his first car and as we were driving along George's Street in Dun Laoghaire, Aiden noticed two friends of Maura's and himself who had been Mater Nurses and now working in The Cedars Hospital which was a T.B. hospital at that time, later to become a Trauma Rehabilitation Centre.

He stopped and asked them if he could give them a lift, which they did not need. I was introduced to both girls one Miss Farrell and the other Eileen Brennan.

A very short time before I left Jervis Street', Aiden invited me to a party in the nurses' home in Monkstown Hospital where he was still working. I gratefully accepted and arrived there on the night. As I had worked two weeks locum for Aiden there I knew many of the staff. There were other junior doctors from St Michael's and nurses from the Cedars also present and I recognised one of the girls that Aiden and Maura had introduced to me in July. I asked her to dance and 'the rest is history'. She was going home to Cork the next day for the New Year and I said I would ring the 'cliché' which rarely happens but it did happen this time when I phoned Eileen on her return from Cork.

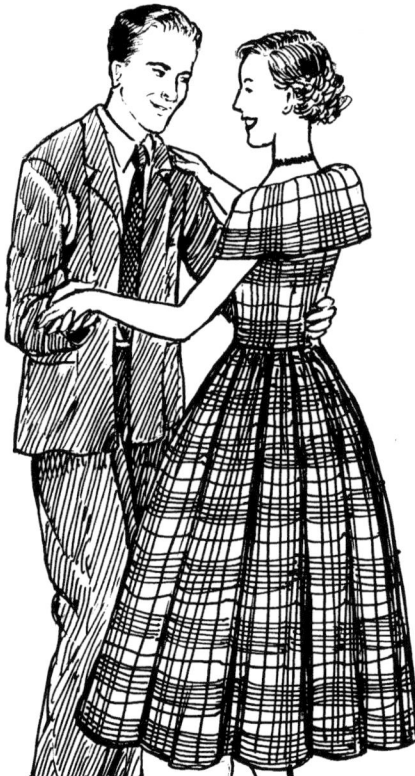

From Slyne Head to Malin Head, A Rural GP Remembers.

In January 1954 we started what was then called 'doing a line' which in 21st century speak is a 'Relationship with or without space'!

It was now a really brilliant time for us all. Eileen and Maura were in the Cedars, Aiden in Monkstown and I was installed in St Michael's with the grand title of Senior House Physician and all within walking distance from each other and for good measure one car. All situated in a beautiful airy place beside the sea and no such thing as pollution. There were short trips to Bray for dinner dances in The Arcadia. Dancing in the famous Top Hat just down the road from Monkstown and walks on the East and West piers.

As there was only one Houseman in Monkstown and as I had frequent off time in St. Michael's I frequently did duty there for Aiden. Eileen and myself used to eat frequently in the restaurant in the Adelphi Cinema in George's Street and we have great memories of the wonderful plaice and chips, which we enjoyed immensely.

At this stage Aiden and Maura were engaged and on the 4th of April 1954 Eileen and myself became engaged and had decided to get married eventually.

During that summer I renewed acquaintance with the light keepers. The Irish Lights Headquarters were situated in Dun Laoghaire area and Monkstown was their official hospital and where they were looked after when required by the staff there. An ex-patient who was a Senior Naval Officer on the crew of the Irish Lights Ship 'Isolda' invited Aiden and friends to visit the ship in the harbour so we all went on board for a very pleasant and interesting afternoon.

The Grand Tour

Another great memory from that summer was a trip that I suggested and was taken on by unanimous agreement and that was a weekend trip to Ballyconneely for the four of us. The plan was to travel in Aiden's car as far as Galway on the Saturday and stay the night there. We booked into the old Imperial Hotel in the square and then on Sunday headed for Ballyconneely via Clifden. Needless to say I was the pilot and guide. We arrived at our destination as arranged for lunch to find my mother at the end of her tether at meeting what could have been her future daughter-in-law who was also screwed up knowing that she was meeting her future mother-in-law. As a 'thaw' gradually set in we enjoyed the lunch and well into the afternoon continued our grand tour of Connemara.

We took the scenic route to Roundstone then on to Ballynahinch Castle Hotel and from there back to the main Galway Road where we turned left towards the Maam Valley and on to Cong and Ashford Castle to mosey around some of the grounds taking photographs and viewing the vastness of Lough Corrib. We then left Connemara and headed back to Galway to get on the Dublin road and back to Dun Laoghaire, well into daylight on the Monday morning. It was a fantastic trip and a wonderful memory.

While all these social activities were going on I was also working in St Michael's where all the house doctors got on very well and we certainly enjoyed our time there. As time went on I was thinking about the future and still considering specialising in medicine. The surgical registrar Rory Lavelle and myself used to have discussions about the future and one day he gave me a textbook on Pathology, which he had used for his Primary Fellowship Exam.

I took it to my room and began to read it that night but fell asleep and when I woke up in the morning all notions of specialising had vanished and I then made the final decision to be a G.P.

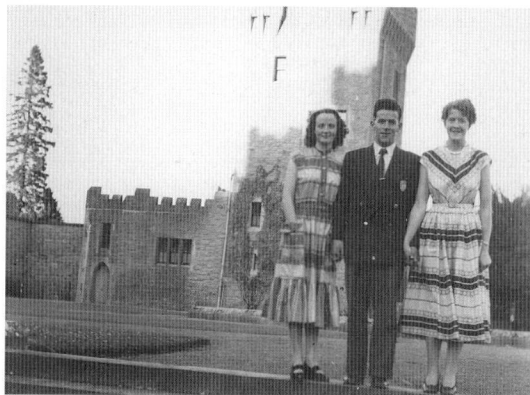

Maura, Aiden and Eileen at Ashford Castle.(1953)

Pilgrims Progress

On another occasion during a meal time in St Michael's, Rory suddenly asked all present if anyone wished to accompany him on a trip to Lough Derg. My mother used to go there frequently with one of her sisters and some friends and I was always intrigued by her stories of the 'tortures and torments' that people suffered while there so I jumped at the invitation to experience this place for myself.

Similar to my first trip to Croagh Patrick I had very little sleep the night before we left as I was on call and up most of the night. This was a bad start as there is no sleep on the first night in Lough Derg and none the next day either. We travelled by train from Dublin I have no idea where we got off the train as I was sleeping before it halted it was probably Bundoran or it may have been Pettigo.

The last part of the journey was by bus so eventually I was in Donegal for the first time in my life and was not impressed with the scenery, which was bleak and dreary.

The next and last time I was to be in Lough Derg was with Eileen shortly before retiring when we had just a short car journey to travel. That was the summer of Italia 90 and we were in Lough Derg the evening that Italy put Ireland out of the World Cup with Scalachies goal in the quarterfinal. Many of us pilgrims were endeavouring to peep through the windows in the staff quarters to get a view of the T.V.

My mother was telling the truth about her experiences. It was a tough exercise going around on sharp stones in bare feet, fasting except for bits of dry bread with Lough Derg soup which was either black tea with pepper or warm water with pepper, whichever it was the cuisine was poor. As regards the weather the Pilgrim was always on a loser. If it was cold it was very cold and if it was warm you were devoured by midges and if it was raining you were really miserable.

The pilgrim got a bed on the second night and there was a traditional story that as the pilgrim stepped into bed he or she would be asleep before lying down. Speaking from experience this phenomenon was a regular occurrence for general practitioners but the big difference was that the G.P. could be called out half an hour later. In Lough Derg there was none of that.

The night's sleep was guaranteed until the big bell rang in the morning and you woke up convinced that you were just slipping into bed so you got very confused not knowing whether you are coming or going but the bell soon leaves you in no doubt. Like Jervis St I enjoyed my time in St Michael's. It was not as hectic or as busy as Jervis St but I was still consolidating my medical experience and it was there that I decided which medical path I would follow.

Monkstown

When the time came in July 54 to leave St Michael's I was certainly not sad as I was only moving down the road to Monkstown to take over Aiden's job as he was moving to The Coombe to do a CC job for three months. Eileen was still in the Cedars so we were all set for another year as I did a locum for Aiden there in July 53 and covered for him several times from St Michael's. I really had a great head start knowing the staff and the routine there.

Monkstown was a very small hospital with a very large through put of patients particularly out patients and minor casualties. Dr. De Courcey Wheeler and his son Desmond who was an Anaesthetist managed the hospital. The Consultant Surgeons, Physicians, Psychiatrists, Radiologists visited Monkstown from other hospitals like Baggot Street, The Meath, Mercers and the Adelaide and there was one junior or hospital doctor who did a bit of everything. It was the ideal type of hospital for general practice training especially after gaining considerable experience in Jervis St and St Michael's.

There was a huge casualty for the size of the hospital and every morning all types of minor accidents and emergencies were seen by a nurse and the houseman. The houseman frequently assisted at surgery in the theatre. Victims of fatal accidents were frequently brought to the hospital so that the local coroner usually ordered post-mortem examination. Having seen many of these being carried out in Jervis St the experience was a great help. I usually had the assistance of the hospital porter when doing these tasks.

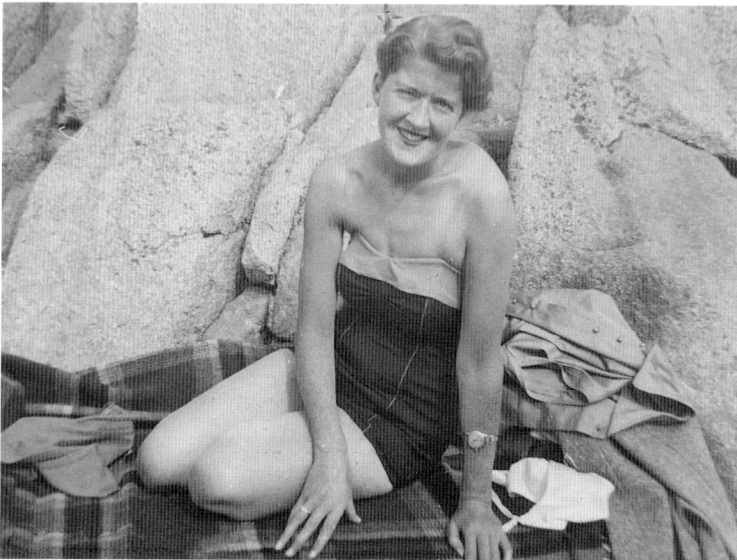

Eileen.(1952)

In those days and well into modern times the official fee for carrying out a post-mortem was three guineas that is three pounds and three shillings and a similar amount for writing a report and attending the inquest to make a total of six pounds and six shillings. At that time it was 'real money' for a junior doctor. There was no regular off time but at odd quiet times I had a quick walk on the west pier. Eileen was free to call into the hospital at quiet times and have a meal in the houseman's sitting room. Fortunately Aiden and Maura frequently covered for a few hours or more so we could get to the Adelphi in Dun Laoghaire to have a meal and see a film or we could have an evening off.

Cork

While Eileen had been to Ballyconneely I had not yet visited her home in Cork so in September 1954 Aiden did a full weekend in Monkstown so that I could travel by train to Cork. Eileen had holidays at that time and was at home in Castlemartyr situated near Middleton between Cork and Youghal. This was a thrilling weekend for me as I had been looking forward to meeting her family.

Her mother was a widow and was a national schoolteacher. Eileen had an older brother Tony and younger sister Margot. Tony was a Civil Engineer and Margot was doing B.Comm in UCC and last but not least a maiden Aunt Eileen who was a wonderful lady and adored by the family. I had a most enjoyable weekend being brought around to view the beautiful beaches and scenery in that area. Now that we had met each others families we were making steady progress.

After finishing his CC job in the Coombe, Aiden had decided to return to UCD to do the Diploma in Public Health (DPH) with a view to obtaining a dispensary job. The plan was to get the DPH in June 55 and then get married so we were all going to be still around until June 55 so he could still relieve me in Monkstown for another year and all of us to continue our social lives.

Around November 1954 I decided that I was financially viable enough to consider purchasing a second-hand car so I began studying the small ads in the Evening Mail. After visiting two garages somewhere on the North Quays I eventually fancied a 1948 Ford Prefect ZE 2512. The cost was around £100, well outside my reach, but it had a good hire purchase deal which allowed me to buy it over a two year period.

Both of us had driving licences so this was a huge boost to our social lives for the foreseeable future particularly when the spring of '55 would arrive.

When we had decided to get married back in April '54 we never mentioned it to anybody but in about April '55 we bought the engagement ring and went public but marriage was still along way off somewhere out there in the distance or was it?

For the time being we had our car, we had the ring and enjoyed making trips to the city, going to shows in the Royal and the Capital and various cinemas. 'This was Dublin in the rare auld times'. There were many trips to Killiney Hill, the Vico Road and out to Bray and the Glen O' The Downs.

By June we were drawing near the end of my time in Monkstown. Despite the very hard work and responsibility I really had a great time there and gained priceless practical experience for general practice. The senior medical staff and the nursing staff were all wonderful particularly the Matron. The night superintendent, Eileen Corbett, who with her husband John, became very close friends of the four of us and this friendship lasted for a long time. They were outstanding and lovely people to know. Monkstown like Jervis Street and the Old Coombe have all been demolished to make way for progress.

Aiden finished the DPH in June and then himself and Maura got married and had their reception in Monkstown Hotel – where else?

The Leaving of Monkstown

They then went to work in a hospital in England with a view of returning to Ireland after a year. I left Monkstown on the last week in June to go back to the Coombe in July to do a CC job.

I was off for the last week in June so Eileen and I went off in our car to Ballyconneely. As far as I can remember the weather was fine but that may have been a perception in our blissful state of mind. There was no drizzle in Oranmore or Galway Bay and we had the longest days of the year. We had a lovely time in Ballyconneely that week with swimming in Erriseask and Ailbrack Beaches and Connemara looking its best.

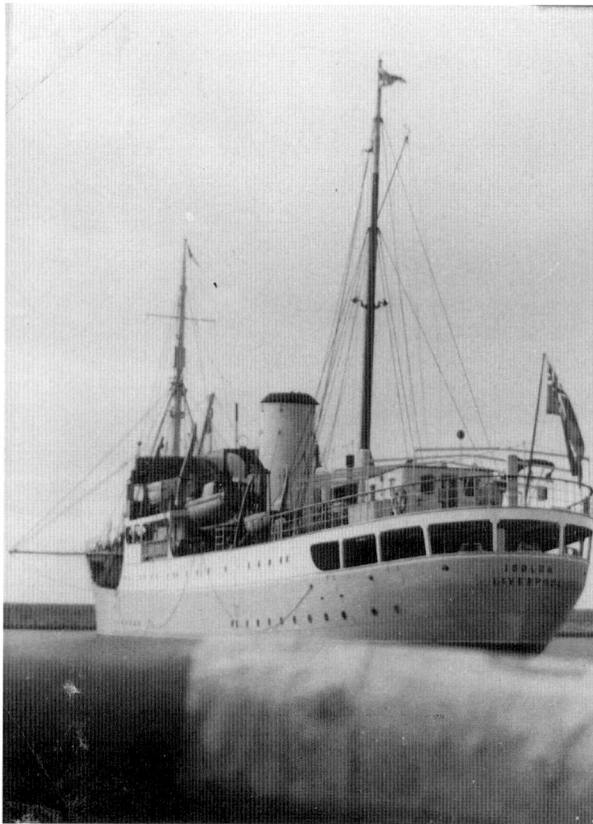

The Light Ship "Isolda", Dunlaoghaire Harbour. (1953)

The Return to the Coombe

On returning to Dublin I went to the Coombe hospital and began the exciting and hectic work of a CC. When there, as a student we had the back up of the CC. This time I was the back up. When I was there, as a student, there was fine weather. This time it was again fine and the start of what was to be a long, hot, exciting and momentous summer for Eileen and myself.

There was a feature about the Old Coombe that all former students and graduates would remember and that was the combination of two distinct aromas that could be experienced in the surrounding air. One was the very pleasant and soothing aroma of malt arising from gigantic vats or whatever in Guinness's and wafting down over the Liffey and in over the Coombe hospital.

The other was the pungent smell of burning flesh or whatever from O'Keefe's the knackers whose establishment was an 'unmarked area' somewhere around. Usually one would be more pronounced than the other depending on the direction of the wind and occasionally they would become mixed to produce some form of a very rare experience that cannot be described. It is possible that the knackers' smell was put there by the hand of God to protect imbibers from becoming overwhelmed by temptation from the aroma of the malt.

From my student days in the Coombe I had built up a good working knowledge of the geography of the large area, which was a great benefit for the driving expertise, required for the CC job. As far as I can remember there were four CCs with a very good rota system two on and two off and alternate weekends off.

The system was a twenty-four hour on twenty-four hour off from 1pm so that you had a morning and evening off every day so that depending on Eileen's time off it was easy to arrange coinciding off time.

With the glorious weather we could frequently swim in Seapoint, which was near Monkstown, which was not yet polluted, also Dollymount (Bull Island). We went once to Killiney but we found it extremely cold. In those days of that memorable summer we had great times. We have a great memory of a sweltering Sunday when we had arranged to go off for the whole day and have a picnic on Portmarnock Strand. After an early start everything went according to plan to make that another great memory. We were having such a lovely time we gave very little thought to our future plans but when August arrived we began to think.

All during my college days I never considered staying in Ireland. I used to read the ads in the British Medical Journal and I had dreams of going to Barbados, America,

Canada and Australia, which would be easy at that time. While I had the greatest respect and admiration for dispensary doctors, I had very strong objections to the system as it existed in the forties and fifties. While they had a steady salary, holidays with pay, and eventually a pension, if they survived, it was amazing that there was no provision for days off or a rota system with colleagues.

Now that we had to make long term decisions we decided to follow Aiden and Maura and go to England and get jobs in NHS Hospitals and after a short time get married. I still had six weeks to complete the Coombe job. Around mid-August two incidents occurred in the Coombe. The first suddenly changed the whole course of our lives. The second could have ended mine.

The First Incident

THE PENNY THAT DROPPED

The first incident occurred one morning as I walked along the footpath, outside the Coombe Hospital, to buy cigarettes (given up in 1959) I met an acquaintance that had been a year senior to me in UCD. We got into conversation and he informed me that he had been doing a locum job in Derry and from there moved into private practice in County Donegal on the shores of Lough Foyle eighteen miles north of Derry in the Inishowen Peninsula. As he was finding the work very strenuous he decided to give up G.P. and take up Public Health Medicine with a nine-to-five day. He had planned to go to UCD to do the Diploma in Public Health (DPH).

As he had built up a substantial private practice he did not wish to walk out without obtaining a replacement. He had decided to make a few enquiries with postgraduates in the Coombe and possibly find one anxious to take it over. He informed me that this was really a long established practice but that young doctors came and went away after a few years. He described Moville as a small town literally on the shores of Lough Foyle in the Inishowen Peninsula and that the large rented house that he was about to vacate would be available for his successor. He also informed me that while he was not really selling the practice, he hoped to get a nominal sum of money to cover the expense of leaving an equipped surgery and waiting room.

I naively thought that when word got around many doctors with more money and experience than me would be offering more money than I had so I told him that I would make enquiries around the hospital. He was on his way to his parent's home for a short break and he walked back with me to the hospital and then gave me his phone number and went on his way.

A short time later a colleague CC who knew the acquaintance asked me where he was working. When I told him the story the reply was – 'Ah Ah' the practice can't be up to much if he is leaving it. At that moment the penny dropped and I thought 'here is the perfect set-up for Eileen and myself and nobody else is interested so that was the last time I mentioned it in the hospital'.

That evening I told Eileen and she immediately replied 'go for it'. I then phoned the acquaintance and asked him if he found anybody interested and he said no. I then informed him that we were very interested. He then invited me to come and stay for a weekend with his wife and himself before making a definite decision. I accepted their kind invitation. We were so excited that we thought this had to be a dream and that we would soon wake up. In our initial excitement and euphoria we had to come back to reality and initiate the process of getting the car over the border which was like getting into the Kremlin in those days. The first procedure was to join the A.A., which was of great assistance in sorting out the required maze of forms and gobbledegook. We took all this in our stride and it added to our excitement at the sudden liberation of no more applications for jobs, no more interviews.

Having become a member of the A.A., I got their advice on the roads to take and they supplied detailed journey maps of the recommended routes to Derry and through the city to Moville. I had arranged the weekend that I would undertake the journey for the first time, which was to be a journey of destiny, which would be travelled on numerous occasions through thick and thin for almost fifty years.

JOURNEY OF DESTINY

On a sunny Friday morning around the 14th of August 1955 I set off from Coombe and headed for Moville taking the road to Drogheda, Dundalk, Castleblaney, Monaghan and a few miles on being checked for the first time at a Customs Post near Emyvale. As the old prefect was burning oil by the gallon I stopped at a garage in Emyvale to top up the oil. As this was a hot day and I could see nobody around it appeared to be 'Siesta Time' so after a short wait I 'mosied' into the garage and looked around but nobody appeared. Eventually I noticed a tin of oil on a shelf marked one shilling and nine pence so I left the required payment, took the tin of oil and topped up the engine with oil and went on my way to cross the border for the first time at Aughnacloy. The names of all the small towns were new to me.

Having gone through the small town of Ballygawley it was on to the well-known town of Omagh, from there to Newton Stewart, then through Sion Mills and into Strabane where I had arranged to meet Charlie.

I had got clear instructions how to find his new house, which I did without any trouble and found him in his usual optimistic and cheerful form. His wife Nancy was in the local hospital, in the early stage of labour with their first child.

He was delighted that I was on my way to Moville informing me that it was a delightful place and that I could not go wrong there. This was great encouragement to make me wonder more and more if I was dreaming. I then carried on through Strabane on the last thirty-one miles to my destination. I soon had my first sight of the River Foyle where the Finn and Mourne Rivers join.

I continued on the main road within sight of the Foyle and the Hills of Donegal in the distance, through the small towns of Ballymagory, Magheramason, and New Buildings alongside the historic river as it flows through the ancient city of Derry. On reaching the famous double-decker metal Craigavon Bridge I took a left turn on the bridge across the Foyle to its western bank then through the city to leave as the river widens to form Lough Foyle until it joins the sea at Inishowen Head.

In a very short time I had reached the Donegal border with two customs posts one on either side of the river that forms the border. At the customs posts in those days it was necessary to get out of the car and take your documents into the hut to have them scrutinised and then your passbook stamped. The Northern Ireland hut was in the townland of Culmore in County Derry. I then drove the car a few yards across the bridge to the southern hut, which was in the townland of Muff, Co Donegal. These documents included the number of the engine and of each tyre on the car. All the customs posts were closed at night so that it was illegal to cross without a special permit after a certain time. As the E.U. developed, all this system gradually disappeared.

I was now in the Republic on the last leg of my exciting odyssey on a glorious August afternoon. I was now in the Inishowen Peninsula and travelling along the shores of Lough Foyle.

After a short distance the beauty of the Lough struck me with the evening sun shimmering on the tranquil blue sea.

While driving slowly I suddenly noticed what appeared to be a town away in the distance situated on a slope going down to the Lough and with a long white wall in the background
.

I got out of the car and up on a ditch to get a better view and suddenly began to wonder if in fact I was looking at Moville. I then got the road map and checked it to confirm that my hunch was correct.

On that hot afternoon I vowed that I would stay in this place and never leave it. Despite many 'hairy trips' in cars through snow and ice, on backs of tractors around the hills of Glackmore, Iskaheen, Crehennan, Glentogher, Glenagiveney, Balleighan etc, etc I never wavered because I knew that the good summers would always turn up. After this exciting interlude I continued on to Moville to find that we could be living in James Street Moville about fifteen yards from the shore of Lough Foyle with the sloping back drop of the recreation green and the white wall.

I got a very warm welcome to Moville from my acquaintance and his wife and after a meal went out with him to do some calls and see some of the countryside. The next day we continued our discussions and instructions while doing calls and being introduced to patients as their incoming doctor. I took several photographs so that Eileen would get some idea of where we were going.

On that Saturday night Jack Duffy the manager of the National Bank as it was then called came on a visit. He had been informed by my acquaintance that he was leaving and had mentioned my name as a probable successor. The manager then asked him where I came from and he replied from somewhere in Co Galway. When I was introduced to him his first question was 'what part of Galway are you from?' When I replied Ballyconneely, Clifden he immediately asked me if I was a son of Tom O'Flaherty.

When I replied yes, he was amazed and told me that he had worked in the National Bank in Clifden around 1918 and that my father had a motorbike on which they both travelled to local functions etc. They were both single at the time. This was indeed a strange coincidence following my chance meeting outside the Coombe hospital. The manager and my father were to meet again in Moville.

Before returning to Dublin we had arranged the change over details, which would be very smooth as the dates fitted our plans perfectly. He was due to start in UCD in early October and my term in the Coombe ended around that time.

On meeting Eileen on the Tuesday we agreed that we would have the wedding in the summer of 1956 and that we would fix the date in a short time. We were now about to start looking around furniture shops.

The Second Incident

THE BACK SEAT DRIVER

One day, a short time after my trip to Donegal, I was off duty and enjoying the sun in the hospital quad when one of my CC colleagues got an emergency call to Inchicore and invited me to accompany himself and a student in this case as it was a haemorrhage I jumped into the back and we took off out the gate at high speed heading for Inchicore with a sharp turn left and then a turn right down Meath Street and on to Thomas Street and James Street. At this stage the ambulance was swaying at a frightening pace so I had great difficulty in holding on to the stretcher beds while the instruments in the big metal box were rattling at a fierce rate.

I appealed to the driver to slow down or we would all be killed or injured as well as the unfortunate woman losing her life.

In my mind there wasn't the remotest possibility of avoiding a crash and had visions of double-decker buses from Inchicore and Kilmainham coming down the hill at Mount Brown and if we met one of them we were 'goners'.

At this stage a man on a bicycle came out a side street and swerved to avoid a stray dog. Our driver then had to swerve and went across the street grazing a wall and then out of control crossed back to the other side and crashed into a lamppost. During this time there was mayhem in the back with numerous obstetric instruments, the metal container and bottles of drip fluid flying around the place.

When silence suddenly returned, I was sitting propped up against the lamppost and feeling dazed, having been pitched out between the two front seat occupants, through the windscreen space, rolled along the bonnet on to the road, with only a broken nose and a superficial graze on one thigh and torn trousers. A corporation Fire Brigade, ambulance and a clergyman about to administer the Last Rites all seemed to have appeared out of nowhere. We reassured everyone that we did not require the Last Rites and requested the ambulance men to take us back to the Coombe. When the ambulance arrived at the door of the gynaecology department two nurses arrived wheeling a trolley to behold three male doctors bleeding and dishevelled. They got into fits of laughter when we reassured them that there was no female patient on board and we did not require any obstetric or gynae treatment this time. The driver went out immediately with another CC to attend the call. All was well that ended well

Floating on Air

The long hot summer of '55 was still going on and Eileen and myself were enjoying it more and more. As we were floating on air and still coming to terms with our good fortune at having grasped an opportunity that was going to map out our future. She had now left the Cedars and was going to work in the brand new St Luke's Cancer Hospital in Rathgar.

In September we went off in the prefect to Cork to give the family a full and detailed briefing on our good fortune and giving glowing descriptions of Inishowen and Moville and reassuring them all that despite the long distance between Cork and Moville we were still in the same country.

As the arrangements about the house in Moville was that my predecessors were moving all the furniture of the private part of the house but leaving the waiting room and surgery furnished. I went on my own to Ballyconneely to give the family a briefing on our good fortune and plans and also to see what bits of furniture I could scrape up from old pieces that I knew had been lying in a store. These consisted of an old iron bed, a broken down chest of drawers and necessary bedding. I arranged for these to be sent by public transport to arrive in Moville before the changeover.

As September was running out rapidly we were coming to terms with being separated for the first time since we met but we were very happy in the knowledge that it would only be a matter of months. As Eileen had not yet been to Moville we planned a visit at the New Year.

As I had a weeks leave from the Coombe, I had arranged to take off the last week and have a week in Moville before the changeover.

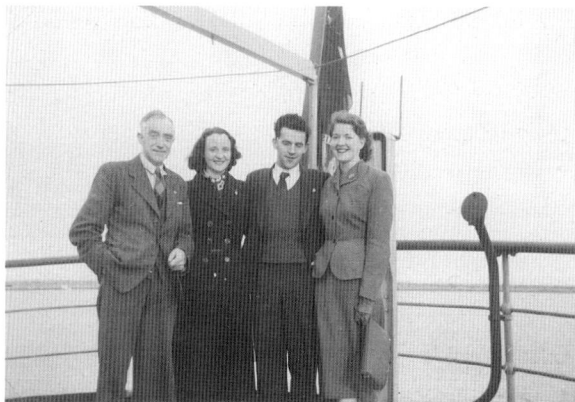

Mr Lally, Maura, Aiden and Eileen touring light ship Isolda. (1953)

The Longest Day

On Monday morning 27th September 1955, the day after an All Ireland final between Kerry and Dublin I packed the prefect with all my worldly goods and chattels.

While at this task a colleague asked me where I was going and when I told him about my destination and plans he said 'Good Luck Boy' with about as much enthusiasm as if I had told him I was heading 'single handed for the South Pole'.

I got into the car and out the gate to leave Dublin for 'the last of the rare aul, times' between Castleknock, UCD, and the hospitals, Jervis Street, the Coombe, St Michael's and Monkstown, I had been fifteen years there. Despite ups and downs I enjoyed it all and had the good fortune to meet my future wife Eileen and made many friends. I was now looking forward to returning to a rural life and a whole new experience.

On leaving the city behind, I was enjoying the views of the countryside on the road to Drogheda. As I approached the top of a hill on the outskirts of the town the prefect began to stall and I got that sinking feeling of trouble.

I was consoled by the fact that if I reached the top of the hill I could 'freewheel' down the other side to reach a garage known as The Black Bull and this was exactly the outcome as the prefect came to a sudden halt on the forecourt and I explained my predicament. The car was parked inside and after the usual questions and superficial examination of the engine etc there was no evidence of the problem so I was informed it would now take a while to sort out.

I then went for a walk but when I returned there was still no sign of a solution to the problem. I then walked into the town and purchased the newspaper to read the reports of the All-Ireland of the previous day and had a cup of tea and buns and then returned to the garage to hear that the problem was not found. As time moved on I kept walking in different directions until lunchtime came and went and still no solution.

After walking several miles more, consuming more tea and buns and having read the Evening Herald, closing time was rapidly approaching and as far as I was concerned crisis time was creeping all over me. My financial situation was in no state to provide staying the night in Drogheda.

As in all good westerns 'The Cavalry' suddenly appeared over the hill as most of the mechanics had gone home and the proprietor in a state of triumph called me to inform me that he had just solved the problem, which was caused by a mass of carbon blocking the exhaust system due to excess burning of oil. Punching a hole with a big screwdriver in the exhaust solved the problem. I was only charged a token fee and in a state of high elation, I drove into the sunset through Drogheda in a thunderous noise belching out poisonous fumes of carbon monoxide in showers of sparks.

In those days cars were not allowed to cross the border without a special pass after a certain hour so I would be too late reaching Muff Customs Post so I decided to change my plans and phone my acquaintance to inform him that I would not be arriving until the next day. I also phoned Charlie and Nancy informing them that I would stay with them that night. I remember making both calls from a coin box in Omagh.

I completed the journey the next day to begin learning the geography of the area. On the following night the 29th September I was with my acquaintance on an obstetric case and delivered my first of many babies in the area.

It became well known that he was the first. He grew up in Moville and went to the National School with two of our sons. He was fondly known as 'Roper'. He became a skilled racehorse rider and rode many winners at local race meetings. He was also a skilled soccer player and played senior football for Sligo Rovers, Dundalk, Derry City and Finn Harps. The next few days passed and on Monday the 3rd October 1955 my predecessor and wife moved out as arranged with all their furniture and I was now in full time single-handed G.P. practice and it was certainly a great help to have had such a smooth change over.

Inishowen Peninsula

Inishowen Peninsula lies between Lough Foyle on the east and Lough Swilly on the west. Strictly speaking Inish is the Irish word for island and Lough is the Irish word for lake. It is probable that in ancient or pre-historic times the ocean could have covered part of the peninsula making it an island. Inishowen as the crow flies is roughly twenty-three miles north to south and twenty-one miles from east to west. There is an official scenic drive around the peninsula called 'The Inishowen 100' (miles).

Malin Head in the north-western part of the peninsula is the most northerly point in Ireland. It is a wild and rugged place but very scenic. It is possible to drive up a steep winding road to the actual head where there is still standing an old watchtower. The highest part of the head is known as 'Bamba's Crown'. Depending on the weather the coast of part of Scotland and some of the isles including the Mull of Kintyre appear just a short distance away.

Lough Swilly and Lough Foyle are beautiful areas but it would be difficult to describe the differences but the fact that the English for Lough Swilly is 'The Lake of Shadows' and this could be the difference. Both have historic pasts…the Swilly from the Flight of the Earls and the Abduction of Red Hugh O'Donnell from Rathmullan, the Foyle for the Siege of Derry and Colmcille's journey by open boat to exile in Iona.

Buncrana is the largest town and has both a seasonal resort trade and a long history of textile manufacturing which like many other areas is having very difficult times.

Carndonagh situated in the centre of the peninsula is the main market town and has a modern district hospital and one of the largest secondary schools in the country and as would be expected a large cattle market and co-op store.

Moville had a bit of everything. Similar to Buncrana it was and still is a hinterland of Derry and during the summer holidays many Derry families rented houses in the town and surrounding areas.

Large numbers of day-trippers came throughout the summer months and smaller numbers come in autumn and spring. In the early part of the last century Paddle Steamers plied between Derry and Moville until the buses took over.

There was always a small amount of fishing in Moville but a much larger amount in nearby Greencastle but with gradual enlargement of the pier and deepening of the harbour Greencastle is now a very large fishing port which is complemented by the adjacent National Fishery College and from the summer of 2002 accommodates the terminal of the car ferry across the Foyle from Magilligan to Greencastle.

Returning to the textile industry there was a large 'cottage industry' of shirt-making by women in the rural areas of Inishowen and this was still going on when I arrived in 1955. There was a shirt factory in Moville at that time which had begun production in 1947 employing up to fifty or sixty women for most of that time for fifty years until, due to the general decline of the industry, it was eventually compelled to close down. The system with the 'cottage industry' was that the proprietor of the factory supplied the women in their homes with material to hand-make the grandfathers' shirts using an ordinary sewing machine. Older men normally wore these shirts at that time. They were usually a grey colour with a bluish stripe and had no collar. Recently they have come back into fashion but with a lighter material and mostly worn by fashion conscious young men. After a certain length of time the factory proprietor returned to collect the newly made shirts and leave a supply of new material. In the course of my medical rounds I had seen these women at work on many occasions. At present there is a new shirt factory in operation on a different site and gradually building up business.

Doctors and Systems at Work

In those days in the dispensary system there was a dispensary doctor to a certain area of every parish or number of small parishes usually with certain boundaries like townlands and rivers etc. Vacancies were advertised and any doctor could apply (except married women). Single women could apply but as soon as she got married she had to resign and return to private practice.

To succeed in obtaining an appointment a high standard of postgraduate experience and several Diplomas or Certificates would be required so that the doctors with the highest number of points like the CAO would be appointed. He or she was paid a salary, four weeks annual holiday every year and a pension at the age of seventy for those who survived long enough.

In addition the doctor was allowed to have private patients who did not qualify for free treatment.

When this scheme started in the late 19th century or early 20th century it was a good system as it was a guarantee that people entitled to free medical treatment were sure to obtain a doctor when required. In my opinion this system had three glaring drawbacks. The first was the retiring and pension age of seventy. I always thought this to be completely outrageous and I could not imagine myself working all day and many nights at seventy years. The second big draw back was having no arrangements for weekend off time, which would be very simple to arrange.

My third objection was that when a vacancy occurred it was filled by a temporary appointment, which at that time could have lasted for several years and almost invariably the temporary occupant was usually dumped and never got the permanent appointment.

The situation in Moville when I arrived was that there was an elderly dispensary doctor who had been resident there for many years. The area had a tradition of a succession of private doctors going back for many years but in more recent years they did not put down permanent roots and only remained for a few years and then moved on without arranging a successor. Fortunately for me my predecessor had the courtesy to arrange a successor and have a very smooth change over. The problem with some of the predecessors was their wives not settling down.

The Old and the New

In 1955 the new National Health Service in England had been established for seven years and I was convinced, without a shadow of a doubt, that a new service was imminent in Ireland and that Dr Noel Brown's 'mothers and child' scheme was the 'thin end of the wedge' which would bring about this change in a very short time and when it would be established I would be automatically in it. It took seventeen years gestation for the GMS to be born but I had no problem with that as I was very happy with my situation in Moville and I had no intention of ever leaving it. I was here to stay.

As a private doctor there was no definite area in which to work. The geographical situation and the border more or less decided rough boundaries. As Moville was literally on the shore of Lough Foyle and there was a main road from Inishowen Head on the north east of the peninsula that went along the shore up the Foyle to the border. That decided that my area would be along the Foyle for seventeen miles to Muff on the border and inland westward and mostly uphill and down the other side for six to twelve miles forming a rectangle of very roughly two hundred and four square miles. There were originally five dispensary areas on the western side of the peninsula, Fahan, Buncrana, Clonmany, Carndonagh, and Malin. On the eastern side there was just one dispensary doctor and one private doctor both based in Moville. On the retirement of the Fahan doctor his dispensary became amalgamated with Buncrana. Today all doctors work from Modern Health Centres.

In 1955 there was a resident public health doctor who worked from the public health office and a clinic in Buncrana. As T.B. was still rampant at that time the public health doctors were very busy and were working very hard holding T.B. clinics all around the peninsula and also frequently visiting houses where new T.B. cases had occurred. In those days the public health doctors where very helpful to GPs and there appeared to be a good co-operation, which was really necessary to control the scourge of T.B.

J. P.

With all the practices mentioned above and with the help of the public health doctors everything would appear to be nice and cosy but that was not the reality. As in many similar situations throughout the country there was no real county hospital or consultants or obstetricians.

There were two buildings used as hospitals and for surgical operations. There was a small hospital in Lifford where some surgery was carried out and a large house in Letterkenny which was used as a hospital and staffed by a few maternity nurses, a few general nurses and a porter and last but by no means least ONE doctor who was the local dispensary doctor, coroner, obstetrician, radiologist and the porter's assistant when he helped the porter to carry post-operative patients from the theatre to their beds. This man was a fully qualified general surgeon who obtained the master of surgery degree from Queens University. This legendry man was Dr J.P. McGinley who was also an active politician who had been involved in The War of Independence and the Civil War and had been a T.D. in the first Dail.

While coming very close to Neil Blaney senior in a general election in the early fifties, he never made it back to the Dail but took an active part in politics until he retired. I had the experience of hearing him loud and clear on a cold winter's night in Moville during an election campaign. I was not at the meeting but heard every word in my house a considerable distance away. On one occasion I had great difficultly in trying to persuade him to admit a patient who was causing me considerable worry and pressure from relatives. In those days the relatives frequently went over the GPs head and got a local, county councillor to plead with J.P. in their case. They hedged their bets and got a Fine Gael and a Fianna Fail councillor to plead. At that stage J.P. came on the phone to me and enquired what 'bloody' foot does that man dig with anyway? I replied that I had no interest whether he dug with one or two feet at the same time as long as I got him admitted. He did and the man lived.

At that time Inishowen had the advantage of being in the Derry hinterland where real emergencies could be treated in either of the two large hospitals there. Letterkenny was forty-five miles from Moville with very poor roads while Derry was twenty miles away and provided out patient treatment for public patients at a very nominal cost of two shillings and sixpence to five shillings. Some of the consultants in Derry had private practices and would come across the border to do private domiciliary consultations if required. This was the situation up to the early sixties when a modern county hospital was built in Letterkenny with a county surgeon, county physician, obstetrician and anaesthetist provided. This was a great leap forward as the facilities in the hospital kept on gradually improving over the years until the present time when it is a large regional hospital with appropriate staff and facilities.

In Derry

The mammoth Altnagelvin Hospital replaced the City and County Hospital and the Waterside Hospital. All down the years the medical staff in Altnagelvin invited the G.P.s of Inishowen to their monthly postgraduate educational meetings. This was a gesture very much appreciated. There was also a similar clinical society in Donegal, which also had a monthly meeting in Letterkenny hospital, which I also attended, but the longer journey on bad roads was time consuming so I attended Altnagelvin more frequently.

New Park and the Montgomery

Similar to many areas around the country since the plantations that have been influenced by certain names like the Eyres of Galway, Moville had the Montgomerys who would have been more familiar in modern times because the name of one of the family who lived in Moville, was none other than Field Marshall Bernard Montgomery of Alamein.

When I came to Moville in 1955 the name was familiar among some of my elderly patients who had been employed in New Park the family home and one was still living in the mews at that time.

There were several generations of Church of Ireland clergymen in the family and Maud Farrer, a daughter of a clergyman, at the age of seventeen, married a clergyman and they had a large family, which included the Field Marshall. His father became a bishop and served in India and Tasmania. He was eventually knighted so Maud became Lady Montgomery. When they retired they came back to New Park and after the Bishop's death she lived there alone until her death in 1949.

She loved New Park and appeared to get on well with the local people. She was a very keen bridge player.

When petrol was not available during World War 2 she used a pony and trap for transport, which reminds me that we also used a pony and trap that time in Ballyconneely. The Field Marshall also loved Moville and returned when possible for short breaks.

New Park was sold and run very successfully as a hotel for several years. When the owners retired it was again sold and changed hands a few times. It became vacant for a long time and very sadly it is now derelict.

The Montgomery family seem to have good relations with the people of Moville and the beautiful recreation green was given to the people provided that no houses would be built there. There is a terrace on the sea front in Moville called Montgomery Terrace.

Property owners had to pay rent to the family, as they were the landlords. As a result of the land acts after Irish Independence there remained a very small rent on property and the Montgomery name was on the official deeds. My rent was four pounds per year.

Early Days

When my predecessors departed my first move was to install the iron bed and the broken-down chest of drawers. Apart from the waiting room and the surgery there was no other furniture apart from a Rayburn cooker in the kitchen. I also had a young, pleasant housekeeper, Mary McLaughlin, who cooked, cleaned and answered the phone and took messages. At that time the phones were on manual exchanges.

During my few days of introduction to the practice I had been introduced to the local midwife and district nurse who were always very helpful. I was also introduced to the two chemists in the town, Charlie McLaughlin and his assistant Hugh Hannon, the other chemist Mr Bennet and assistant Dympna Cooke (later O Donnell). I was introduced to the owner and son of a very important facility the local garage. Joe the owner and son Lawrence who promised they would never see me stuck, and are still keeping their word forty-five years later in the hands of grandson, Michael.

On the third day I attended my first delivery with the midwife it was also the first baby for the mother. In those days and for many years to come there was no special off time for GPs. My predecessor had developed a system of taking short breaks on a Wednesday as that was the half-day in the town and I continued the system. It was not a prefect arrangement but at least it helped. As a private doctor I had not signed contracts so the 'buck' stopped with the dispensary doctor. As the planned system at that time never had, or never contemplated having, a built in weekly off time or breaks. I never contemplated taking up golf as I always had visions of being called away as I teed up at the first green or about to hole a putt to win the captain's prize.

In the early days, on my own, I usually took a few hours off and explored around Derry or visited the other small towns in Inishowen or venturing as far as Letterkenny, or just driving to a quiet place and having a sleep in the car.

When the mother and child scheme became official, private doctors were involved and got paid by the health service for attending most maternity patients and contracts were signed. When away I now phoned home more frequently and I had a good back-up from the midwife. As mentioned previously I was very pleased with this scheme as I was certain that a new general scheme with a choice of doctor had to be near. At that time there was another advance to the choice of doctor and that was in allowing private doctors to certify severely disturbed psychiatric patients to a psychiatric hospital. There is a new mental health act due for many years but has not yet arrived.

Doing it My Way

In 1955 very few GPs worked appointment schemes. Even then working without appointments was not efficient but I could not contemplate rushing to keep up to the appointments. This may have been due to my training with Dr Billy O'Dwyer who spent a long time obtaining a detailed history from the patient and then did a very thorough and slow examination. I always felt more relaxed with this system rather than rushing. I had this obsession that I could never keep up with the appointments and that tension would build. I even had a built in system in myself that when the large waiting room became crowded I automatically slowed down and that weeded out the patients with trivial complaints and eventually left the more serious patients.

As rural GPs. always had to deal with minor or severe casualties, chiefly lacerations, where minor surgery was required it could not be rushed. How did a lone GP cope with a six-inch gash full of gravel, tend to it and still see the next patient on time? It succeeded in evacuating half of the crowded waiting room. And that's how? When I eventually had a full time practice nurse to assist me it certainly improved my speed but I still had the in-built slow pace. I accept that everything has speeded up and that in modern times appointments systems are necessary.

When I first started I had the same surgery hours as my predecessor, which was from 1:30 to 3:30 pm and 7:00 to 8:00 pm, and doing outside calls in the morning and more after the afternoon surgery. This went on for several years with the 3:30 pm surgery becoming longer and longer until it ran into the 7:00 to 8:00 pm night surgery, which gradually went on to late at night when eventually men were arriving after the pubs closed and women after the pictures! I then cut out the night surgery completely except for urgent cases and emergencies and had one surgery from 10:00 am to 4:00 pm with a half hour break for lunch and then did outside calls after 4:00 pm, which usually finished much later. All this went on with emergencies and accidents coming in, so at times it became chaotic. The one thing that maintained my sanity and competence was that I did not or could not rush.

Home Deliveries

In the early days from 1955 until 1962-63 when home births were still the order of the day or more correctly night, doing an average of one per week added to the apparent stress.

I always preferred to attend maternity patients at night because in the middle of the night there was less likely to be a queue of patients in the waiting room or a build up of calls that occurred when delayed during the day so that it took another day and part of a night to catch up on the normal routine. Fortunately most deliveries occurred at night so that returning at around 6:30 to 7:30 am the routine was a wash and shave before breakfast and a start of another day.

This type of experience had some compensation coming home at dawn on a summer morning but crawling home on an icy road in the depths of winter was something else! During those times I really appreciated the great store of practical experience I had built up in the old Coombe. The compensation of attending home births was the great sense of satisfaction at assisting and helping the mothers to achieve a difficult delivery. I always felt more reassured when working with a midwife as they had the same training as doctors and usually more experience.

When I think of the number of elderly dispensary GPs. who carried this burden for their whole career and well into their seventies my mind boggles! They should have got automatic canonisation!

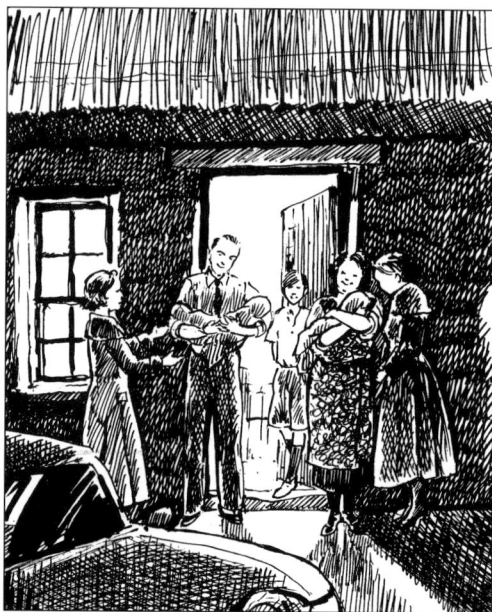

From Slyne Head to Malin Head, A Rural GP Remembers.

And Then There Were Three

During those obstetric years I feel that it is worth recording how we dealt with multiple pregnancies. If twins were suspected during the anti-natal care there were no scans or ultra sounds, or other technology or consultant obstetricians to confirm your 'hunch' so we had to depend on the old x-ray and the patient was sent to J.P. in Letterkenny for the x-ray and who would report his findings directly to the patient to convey the news to the doctor if there was one or two and that was it! So we went on with anti-natal care and nobody died of radiation and eventually twins would be delivered at home. I had this experience four times.

On another occasion I also suspected twins and referred the patient for x-ray. J.P. was as usual very busy but kindly examined the film, and emerging from the x-ray department with the film, he put up two fingers and shouted to the patient to tell her doctor that there were two babies shown on the film.

The pregnancy and anti-natal care went on as usual and when labour started the midwife was called and she advised calling the doctor and when I arrived the mid-wife had delivered a small baby girl, which had appeared normal otherwise.

In the traditional technology of the day for very small babies she was wrapped in cotton wool and we awaited number two but after no sign of it we eventually, without going into details, extracted the 'second' twin and then to my consternation I found another one to bring the grand total of three tiny little girls all just under three pounds weight all wrapped in cotton wool. The mother was none the worse, the midwife and myself were shattered but very happy sharing the excitement that now erupted in the household and spreading like a bush fire around the neighbours.

I got on the phone to Letterkenny to enquire from a maternity nurse if they had an incubator, which they had, and they would be delighted to take care of the triplets until they were strong enough to return home. At that stage I had recently purchased a new Ford Anglia (with a heater) so I drove up and down the main road until it was well heated and then got the mid-wife and a few neighbours with the stars of the moment, the triplets, and headed for the forty five miles to Letterkenny to hand them over to the midwives in the hospital who did a magnificent job in looking after them until they were strong enough to return home.

On that day of their births I realised that I had an experience that by the laws of averages would never be repeated but we all know now that in the world of technology the odds are now much shorter due to fertility pills and advancing technology. The girls grew up, eventually got married and had families.

The First Christmas

To return to autumn 1955 and my early experiences I was still finding my way and by Christmas I had a working knowledge of the roads and district thanks to the great help I received from many people giving advice and directions. I was invited by the Duffy family to have Christmas dinner with them. I was entertained by Jack recalling his life and probably 'half' of his experiences in Clifden and Ballyconneely.

I enjoyed this very much but I would never be a nostalgic or home sick. As was the norm for GPs in those days I was on call and shortly after the dinner I got a call and several more for the remainder of the day. I had worked the previous Christmas in Monkstown and had a rushed dinner in the nurses dinning room. I was destined to work for twelve more Christmas days until we got the first rota system going in 1968

Love Letters

Needless to say that during these three months, letters were flying between Eileen and myself. The wedding was by now arranged for the 14th of June 1956 in St Patrick's church in Cork and the reception to be in the Metropole in McCurtain Street. Despite the dreary time of the year we had arranged for Eileen to come and see Moville for the New Year. She travelled by train which came in at the old station on the west side of the Foyle and which is now preserved as a Railway Museum and Heritage Centre with an old Donegal railway engine parked outside the terminal. She stayed in the Prospect Hotel just across the street from our house and overlooking Lough Foyle. Despite the dark days she was very impressed with the whole area.

We arranged that I would make a trip to Dublin in January to attend the annual Mater Hospital dance, which was always a big night in the Gresham Hotel. This was just now a few weeks away so it eased the loneliness of our parting after the few days together. We arranged that I would drive to Dublin the day before the dance and stay overnight and return to Moville on the following day. I was looking forward to this break, as my social life had been very limited during the first three months due to the settling in process.

Let it Snow, Let it Snow, Let it Snow

The day eventually arrived and I went off in the Prefect fortified with a large rug and a fleece-lined airman's leather jacket, which were sold as US Army surplus stocks at bargain prices after the war. We had a most enjoyable night at the dance it was now 1956 and only five months to the wedding.

Eileen was off the next day so we met again and after a meal went to the pictures in the Ambassador before I was due to return to Moville. When we came out from the film it was very cold and there were odd snowflakes flying around. To say the least I was not looking forward to the journey home as I had very little sleep on the night of the dance and I was now feeling very cold and tired. We parted after planning another trip to Dublin in the spring and off I went.

I was certainly glad to have the woolly jacket and the rug which were standard equipment in all cars up to the fifties before car heaters were 'allowed' in this country and I imagine also 'banned' in the U.K. despite the fact that the Americans had them as standard for many years. This reluctance to have heaters was the old conservative myths mentality of the anti-freeze destroying your engine, the radio wrecking your battery and the seat belt causing accidents. When I purchased my first car, a green Anglia in 1957, the dealer informed me that I could have a heater installed for twelve pounds and ten shillings extra. Needless to say I was delighted to hear that we had got into the 20th century at last.

So to get back to the Prefect and the return journey everything went well until somewhere around Dundalk the snow gradually got heavier as I travelled towards Castleblaney but there was no real problem so far with the old Prefect as the older cars were always superior in snow to the modern cars. Despite the bitter cold I was comfortable in the woolly jacket and there was no danger of falling asleep as the risks in snow always concentrated the mind. From around Omagh the snow was building up and I was really worried and hoping that if I could make it to Strabane I would stay the night with Charlie and Nancy.

When I reached the hairpin bends on the Omagh side of Newtonstewart it was worse but at least I was going downhill but to my horror there were diversion signs on the road as there were road works on the bends at that time. This diversion led up a narrow road for about a quarter to half a mile to a T-junction where there was no visible diversion sign as it would be covered in snow which was now building up and I was really terrified and rapidly decided that it was safer to get snowed in on a main road than up a narrow by-road. I managed to turn the car and get back on the main road to take a chance of going down the steep hill and hope against hope that there were no barricades or steep water holes on the way but I was lucky and reached the town so my chances of reaching Strabane were revived and much to my delight the snow got lighter as I went on. When I reached Strabane it had cleared so it was not necessary to bother Charlie and Nancy and I just pressed on to Derry and Moville at a very slow pace on the icy roads and struggling to keep awake.

I now go fast forward many years later during the height of the troubles and with Eileen and myself driving a BMW. I missed seeing a diversion sign on that same road and as we approached the town three police cars surrounded us with sirens blaring and flashing lights.

I remember saying to Eileen we are really in the 'soup' now as there was one RUC man at the front writing the registration number into his notebook, another at the window and another at the back. As I let down the window I did what I always do in these circumstances eat humble pie, apologise profusely and hope for the best.

The man was very nice and civil and urged me to be more observant in the future and to be sure and drive carefully for the rest of the journey.

Rewinding back to January 1956, on reaching home the house was like being in a freezer and all I could do was to take off my shoes and get into bed in all my clothes including the woolly jacket. I imagine I fell into a 'coma' rather than a deep sleep and woke up six hours later in the exact same position as I was in when I lay down. It was a bright frosty morning with the Foyle shimmering in the winter sunlight and I was wondering if the journey home was a dream or a nightmare!

I was now back at work and still coming to terms learning the many different highways and byways, but it was becoming easier very day as everybody was very helpful and I had no difficulty in understanding the dialect which was similar in many ways to west Connemara. My education in the pub, the bogs, the hay fields, tillage and crops and the perpetual Irish topic of conversation the weather made communication very pleasant.

Doctor Gets Married

As the 14th of June deadline was approaching rapidly I made another trip to Dublin in late April and this on serious business as we had to purchase at least some basic furniture. Off I went fortified with an overdraft. We did the business and requested it to be sent to Moville.

The next time we would meet would be in Cork. I had arranged with a UCD classmate to do two weeks locum while we would be away.

The last few weeks were extremely busy and tension was building up rapidly. At the end of May and early June I witnessed for the first time the real long bright evenings in north-west Donegal with no complete darkness on clear nights. Unfortunately this beautiful phenomenon is usually blotted out by rain and cloudy weather conditions. The locum arrived the day before I departed for Cork and I gave him as much information as possible to enable him to find his way around.

I had decided to break the long journey to Cork by staying in Dublin for one night and then completing the journey on the following day, so I headed for Dublin on Sunday the 10th June and completed the journey on the following day.

As was the custom in those days the wedding on the 14th was in the morning so that after the long breakfast we left on our honeymoon in the late afternoon by first driving to Dublin where we stayed for two nights. We went to the latest musical show of the

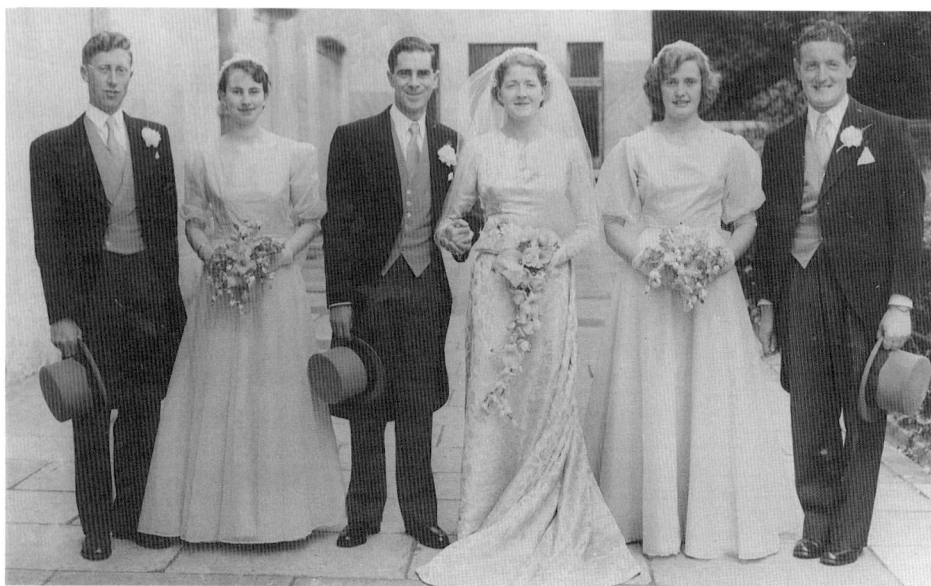

Ken's Marriage to Eileen. (14th June 1956)

From Slyne Head to Malin Head, A Rural GP Remembers.

time Salad Days in the Olympia and on the following day flew to Jersey. The usual custom in those days of the early morning weddings was a mad rush after the breakfast to an airport or boat.

On looking back we were away ahead of out time in our leisurely departure as in modern times the custom is even more relaxed with the afternoon weddings and the couple staying until the next day. Apart from the bumpy flights we enjoyed our trip to Jersey.

On our return to Dublin we stayed for another night before collecting a load of presents which were stuffed into the Prefect and for the one and only time ever we had to take the long route from Dublin to Moville to avoid the customs hassle.

This entailed driving across the country to Sligo and the hundred miles to Moville on the appalling roads of those days. At least we had daylight almost all the way.

On arrival to our home in James Street, Moville that night we had completed a magnificent 'Roller Coaster' which began on that warm August morning ten months previously when we had no set plans and had no idea when we would be married but by grasping an opportunity coming out of the 'blue' by immediately accepting a man's word we were now married, had an established practice and our own rented home situated in a most beautiful place within a few yards of the sea.

The Scottish Fairs

Donegal has an abundance of magnificent scenery including a long coastline of magnificent beaches, bays, mountains, glens, lakes and bog lands. The one drawback which is now being addressed is its geographical situation which apart from the political border appears to be isolated from the rest of the country, but its closeness to Scotland which is only a few miles from Inishowen Head had a very big influence on the whole county.

In the nineteenth and twentieth centuries when thousands of Irish people emigrated to America and Canada most Donegal people went to Scotland to work in the great shipyards in Glasgow where there was huge employment for different crafts. The closeness of the two countries made travel back and over very convenient while many people who went to America never returned.

Up until the late sixties or early seventies there were frequent passenger and cattle boats plying between Glasgow and Derry.

The American liners came to Derry but anchored at Moville to take on passengers from tenders. When we came to Moville, in 1955-56, there were regular boats to Derry and many people from Inishowen and I presume from other parts of Donegal travelled on these ships for short visits to relatives in Scotland.

This closeness led to a tradition in the Glasgow areas of large numbers of workers and families having fixed summer holidays known as Fairs. Different areas closed down for holidays at set times. There was a Glasgow Fair, Greenock Fair and a Paisley Fair (nothing what ever to do with the reverend Doctor in Belfast!).

Many went to local Scottish resorts but huge numbers came to Donegal and particularly to Inishowen. Extra ships were laid on for Derry in June and July and I have vivid memories of several taxi loads of visitors arriving in the early hours to James Street where we lived. This would be usually around 6 am and there would be great activity collecting luggage and going into the Prospect Hotel across the street and to a nearby boarding house. Many houses around the town catered for smaller numbers and there were also many rented houses occupied.

The fairs were a great source of income for many people and for the town in general. Huge numbers of families with relatives in the surrounding district came to holiday with them. As they were all of Irish descent they had a great mixture of Irish and Scottish humour, which changed the whole scene.

As we all know June and July can have very good or very bad weather but bad weather never bothered the visitors but it bothered us locals who felt that there was no hope of good weather until the fairs were over. I was convinced that the weather in Scotland was much worse than other areas so that the visitors appreciated the Donegal weather. There was a perception in the town that the day the first fair arrived a well-known draper would have had racks of plastic coats hanging outside his premises for early morning arrivals!

While driving around a wide area visiting patients I had a sort of bird's eye view of how the visitors always appeared to be enjoying themselves immensely as many groups could be seen in their plastic raincoats in the best of humour as they walked along in the drizzle. The best part of the day had yet to come when the singing in the pubs started. I should know because the Trawlerman (previously Packie's Bar) was beside me and the Prospect across the street.

The fairs were certainly a compensation for the lack of general tourist trade in north Donegal. This brings us back to the geographical situation when the Victorians came to visit Ireland on holiday they appeared to take the short trip to Rosslaire or Dublin to reach the trains which made it very easy to travel west to Killarney or Galway and Connemara and to a much lesser degree to Sligo or Bundoran.

I have vivid memories of the large numbers of tourists to be seen in Connemara every summer in the thirties. The reverse of this theory is that the majority of people emigrating from the west of Ireland went to England while those from Donegal went to Scotland.

The number coming on the fairs began to decline in the early sixties and this trend continued until the Derry boats were withdrawn through the lack of trade and this was a severe blow to the numbers of visitors but the killer blow was the start of the troubles in Derry. As the times were rapidly changing everywhere the demise of the fairs was inevitable
.

I could see this coming before my eyes in the fifties and early sixties when I was very busy during the fairs being called to families in rural areas where visitors, usually with children, would be ill. Over the years these children grew up and when the grandparents died these families went on holiday to Spain so cultural changes also played a part in the demise of the Scottish fairs.

During the fairs and the remainder of the summer months it was usually very busy in the surgery especially with children having minor accidents falling on rocks or lacerations from broken glass and frequent asthma attacks.

The Regatta

Most small towns had some special events in July or August, particularly on the August bank holiday weekend, either a show, or horse races, a fleadh or something. Moville was no exception. As the town was built on a hill near the sea above the beautiful green, which sloped down to the water's edge, it had the prefect setting for a regatta, which was held on the Monday of the August bank holiday weekend. This weekend was also the traditional start for holidays in Derry going back to the days of the old paddle steamers carrying day-trippers to Moville.

As our high two-storey house was situated a few yards from the sea we had a grandstand view of the whole proceedings.

In addition to the Derry day-trippers it was also a day off for the local people from the large surrounding country area.

It was certainly not a day off for me as work gradually increased by the hour due to elderly people collapsing, adults and children with minor injuries filled the waiting room while emergency calls to car crashes were frequent especially at night. I remember many regatta days and nights when I never got to bed.

Around this time there were also smaller regattas at Inishowen Head and Greencastle. As time moved on the Moville Regatta very gradually declined in popularity particularly when the troubles started in Derry and with changing lifestyles. Despite the difficulties it is still surviving.

Sea Angling

One of the big changes in lifestyle that occurred in the mid-fifties was the development of sea angling festivals. This idea was pioneered in Westport, County Mayo. In January 1957 this idea was taken up by a few enthusiastic people in Moville who travelled to Westport that summer to see how it was done there and came back convinced that Moville and Greencastle had the facilities for staging a large festival similar to Westport.

The large number of small trawlers made this possible in Greencastle. The first Moville Sea Angling festival was held on the last week in August 1957. This ambitious plan was very successful and attracted sea angling enthusiasts from northern and southern Ireland and also from the U.K. This week long festival went on for several years but due to changing circumstances it was eventually reduced to two weekends.

Greencastle had gradually became a very large fishing port adjacent to the National Fishery School so the trawlers had become very much larger and there were fewer small trawlers available for sea angling.

During the festival week and later the two weekends there were the usual side shows including large opening and closing ceremonies. When in 1968 I got alternate weekends off I accompanied our sons taking part in the festival, which I enjoyed much more than fresh water fishing. In 1997 the festival celebrated its fortieth anniversary. In more recent years there is also an oyster festival in September, which promotes development of the Foyle Oyster fishing industry.

Bernard's Wedding

In late August 1956 Bernard and Lucy Smith were married in the Church of Christ the King in Salthill Galway and the reception was in the Bamba Hotel.

Lucy was originally from Ballinasloe and had been a nurse in the district hospital in Clifden. Eileen and myself, now an old married couple of two months, enjoyed our trip to Galway and returned two days later.

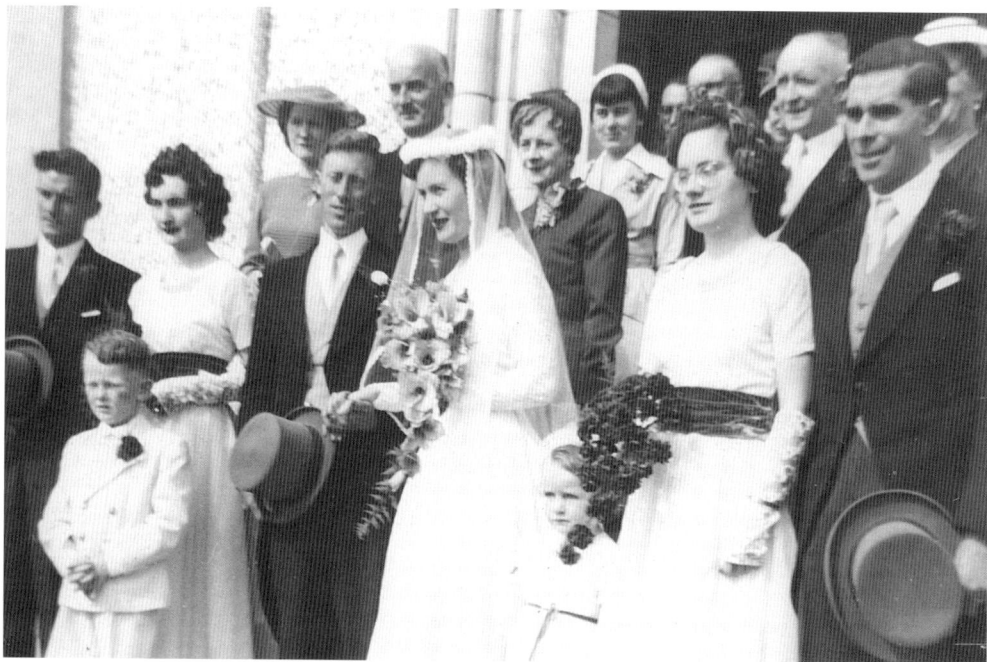

Bernard's Wedding. (1956)

Doctor at Sea

In the fifties and up to the early eighties doctors were frequently called out to attend sick or injured crewmember on trawlers or merchant ships. The trawlers were mostly Spanish or French. The merchant ships could be any size or nationality.

The procedure in the mid-fifties was that all merchant ships and deep sea trawlers had agents in various ports so when injury or illness struck, the captain contacted the nearest agent who then notified the nearest pilot station. He in turn notified the local sub-agent in Moville who informed the doctor to be at the pilot station at a certain time to accompany them in the pilot boat to a rendezvous with the merchant ship or trawler. This could be any agreed point in Lough Foyle as far as the Foyle Buoy just off Inishowen Head.

In the early part of the nineteenth century the pilot boats were under sail and the pilots boarded the sailing ships on the north west of Inishowen. In the fifties the pilot station was a small building with a small landing stage at Inishowen Head when an open boat with an outboard engine was used. After some years the station was moved to Carrickarory Pier on the Derry side of Moville and since 2001 it has a permanent station in Greencastle. From the seventies, the pilot boats were much larger with sheltered facilities and modern equipment and could travel at much faster speeds.

When the pilot boat reached the ship or trawler he manoeuvred along the leeward side where the ladder would have been lowered. The pilot then boarded and the next procedure was to lash the doctor's bag to a rope to be hauled on board then I would climb up the ladder and was assisted over the rail by a member of the crew. Boarding a trawler was no problem as the sides were low. On a big merchant ship the climb was longer on a rope ladder and in very high seas a safety rope was tied around your body so if you did fall it would be simple to get hauled on board. In calm weather an accommodation ladder would be provided and this was similar to the gangway used for boarding large passenger ships in port.

Normally I was not prone to seasickness but on some occasions I could feel queasy and that would be put to the test on French or Spanish trawlers not by the overwhelming smell of fresh fish but by the awful cigarettes smoked by the crews. Despite the fact that that up to 1959 I smoked 'Gold Flake' myself and 'Woodbine' before I reached the use of reason but when I went down below to the sleeping quarters it was almost overwhelming. I reckoned that providing I was in normal health and about to carry out a highly responsible job I could not get sick.

Unfortunately I did not keep a diary or any form of record of the different ships and trawlers I had attended but I can attempt to recall at least some of the experiences I had and observations that I made and also what I had learned.

I rarely attended any patient that was really sick apart from serious accidents caused by seamen falling into holds.

I remember seeing a very ill psychiatric case who was obviously a danger to himself and the crew and the only one I had ever seen constrained in a straight jacket.

I am sure there was a policy that there was no such thing as a crewmember becoming a passenger even for one or two days. I learned very quickly that there was no point in reassuring the captain that the patient had flu and would be well after a few days on aspirins or panadols. The captain's reply was invariably 'No Bono, No Bono, send home or go hospital'. Another experience was not to take the trouble of removing foreign bodies. In this case there was a fish bone stuck in a man's foot and after injecting local anaesthetic and some poking around I removed the bone and gave him antibiotics and reassured the captain that he would be fit after a few days but the reply was No Bono etc etc etc.

I understood this policy very well because if not enforced the captain could finish up with passengers instead of a crew.

This policy also removed a load off my mind when all I had to do in future was to examine the patient and advise sending him home or to hospital. When returning home the sub-agent made all the arrangements.

I learned one hard lesson when I was called to examine the body of a man who had died suddenly on a trawler. After obtaining a detailed history from the captain about the dead man's illness if any before he died etc etc and having examined the body and finding no sign of violence I was satisfied that he had suffered a severe coronary thrombosis (Heart Attack). In those early days post-mortems were a rare procedure in Donegal except in very exceptional circumstances so the local coroner would give a GP. permission to give a death certificate. Having got permission from the coroner I signed a certificate and gave it to the agents to look after the rest of the funeral arrangements.

All went well until the body reached the border and then there were all sorts of confusion because in the northern jurisdiction a death certificate in this case was not valid until a post-mortem was carried out. I was having panic phone calls from the north and south customs, the RUC, the city and county hospital, shipping agents etc which I was pleading all kinds of ignorance and expecting a Black Maria to take me away any moment!

Eventually I was notified by the RUC that the state pathologist in Belfast had been alerted to carry out a post-mortem examination on the body in the City and County Hospital and that I was to be present to witness it on that evening. Needless to say the pathologist found that it was due to a massive coronary thrombosis as well as been proved correct in my diagnosis I had also learned a lesson about sending bodies over the border.

While the language barrier was a small problem when examining patients on foreign ships or trawlers it was still very helpful if an interpreter was available so the main agents in Derry occasionally sent a man from Derry who could speak French and Spanish. Without an interpreter varies signs and gesticulation are carried out for communicating

On one occasion when examining a man with a possible urinary problem I was trying to elicit if he had a pain or difficultly passing urine, I had used every possible sign, gesticulation, pointing at various parts of his anatomy and the only answer I could get was 'no comprehendo, no comprehendo'. Pointing once more to his bladder region, bending myself in two and mimicking great distress and agony, I shouted, 'Can you piss-piss'. His eyes light up and he raised up his two arms shouting 'comprehendo-comprehendo, peess – peess'.

Although in the mid and late fifties the war was long ended there were still U.S. and British naval bases in Derry so that various sorts and sizes of naval ships were frequently anchored in Lough Foyle opposite Moville. These included submarines and the occasional aircraft carrier. On one occasion I was on the pilot boat when it went along side a submarine so I had a close up view of the sub, which struck me as being a dark, and weird looking ship.

Speedy Gonzales

After several trips to French and Spanish trawlers I was amazed at the speed they could turn around and head out Lough Foyle the instant the pilot stepped on to the deck of the pilot boat. Usually I was escorted to the boat followed by the pilot and when I had my two feet on the deck and looked around the trawler would have disappeared, going full steam out the Foyle. I often wondered if one of them ever got away with the pilot still on board.

On a cold Sunday afternoon I witnessed this FEAT. As the boatman revved up the engine somebody suddenly said 'Where is Joe?' (pseudonym). Another pointed to the distant trawler 'There he goes on his way to Spain'. We all had some hilarity imagining which expletive Joe was now using. In fact there was no real problem as he could disembark at Greencastle a short distance away. But the captain would not have been amused at the slight delay to his speedy get-away.

I have memories of boarding a very large Russian fish factory ship off Inishowen Head. It was in the month of June but very stormy for that time of year. I had to examine a man who was very sick with a very acute appendicitis - requiring emergency surgery.

The captain did not wish to go up the Foyle to a more sheltered area but insisted that the patient should be taken on to the pilot boat.

While this feat was taking pace I was invited to have a meal, which I did not enjoy and at the same time watch a black and white war film where the Russian forces were well on top. Eventually the patient, lashed on to a stretcher, was lowered on to the pilot boat to return to Moville and transferred to a waiting ambulance on Carrickarory Pier.

The Moville Record

Another memory in going out to a very large merchant ship bound for the U.S.A. I have no memory of the patient but what I can remember very well is that it was a flat, calm, Wednesday afternoon in September with a dense fog and the plan was to rendezvous with the ship at the Foyle Buoy.

When we reached the area nothing was visible but when we got near the buoy the tinkling of the bell could be heard and the pilot was in radio contact with the ship. The sounds of the bell were reassuring in the weird surroundings of the dense fog.

Eventually while moving very slowly we got alongside the big ship and I began the longest climb I can remember on a rope ladder. This was the one boarding that remained unique in my memory because either the captain or a member of the crew came from a place called Moville in Iowa U.S.A. I did not discover this until two months later a newspaper called the Moville Record arrived in the post with the added title of Official Woodbury County Newspaper dated 4th of November 1971. I discovered later from local people here that they had heard of the twin town. Come to think of it there has to be hundreds of Irish towns named in the U.S.A. but the coincidence of this man on a non-scheduled visit to the area is worth recording.

Force Ten

The roughest night that I can remember on the pilot boat was on a very stormy Saturday night in March. I got the call around 8:00 pm and it was to a very large Swedish merchant ship to attend a crew member who had fallen into a hold and who had multiple fractures on legs and arms. As we left Moville it was blowing a force ten gale, which was not very bad at first but deteriorated as we got near the head and the safety rope was reassuring as I climbed the rope ladder.

When I got to the man still in the hold I was relieved to find that the captain and medics had him very well splinted in the then inflated plastic splints.

He had no compound or open fractures and he had lost very little blood, he had fractures on both legs and one arm and had severe shock and pain so morphine was given. Due to the severe winds he could not be transferred to the pilot boat so the captain requested me to remain overnight on the ship, which would proceed towards Derry but would anchor overnight at Moville.

The conditions in this huge ship were first class. The pilot and myself were entertained to a very good meal and then shown to a very comfortable cabin for the night. I visited the patient twice during the night to administer morphine. In the morning the gales had abated so I disembarked and got back on the pilot boat to the pier to carry on the rest of my weekend on call. The pilot brought the ship to Derry where the patient was transferred to Altnagelvin Hospital.

Joker in The Pack

I can recall one more unusual trip on the Foyle, which occurred on a later phase of my life when Greta, my practice nurse, assisted me. The call came in the early part of the day during a busy surgery. There were no details given so after instructing Greta to keep things going in the surgery as best she could, I went off on another trip on the Foyle on the pilot boat.

There was a much longer than usual wait at the Foyle Buoy for the ship which was in fact a survey ship. I have forgotten the nationality but most of the crew could speak English and their last port of call was some part of Poland where the crew had shore leave and where there was an ample supply of hostesses and escorts. All the crew on shore leave got gonorrhoea. Those were the days when H.I.V or Aids had not yet arrived and the 'living was easy' and a rapid course of sulphonamides did the trick.

The medical orderly on board insisted that I examined every patient. When I had finished the ship's launch was dispatched to the local chemists for a 'load' of sulphonamides. I returned on the pilot boat wondering how Greta was coping and much to my delight she had coped extremely well with the unsolicited help of one of the waiting patients a man who was well back in the queue but determined to make it shorter by frequently going outside and viewing out the Foyle to see if there was any sign of the returning pilot boat and reporting back to the queue that the doctor was now out near Inishtrahull (an island north of Malin Head) and would not be back until night. In actual fact there were no serious emergencies and most of the queue including the joker himself had gone home.

History

While I am writing here about my experiences and events that I have witnessed whether well or otherwise I am recording history.

At present medical emergencies on ships are treated by advice on radio and computers and when hospital treatment is necessary doctors can be lowered from helicopters or patients can be winched up and in a very short time landed on a hospital helipad.

While these trips to trawlers and ships were exciting diversions for me it was a daily routine for pilots and boatmen frequently in very bad weather conditions.

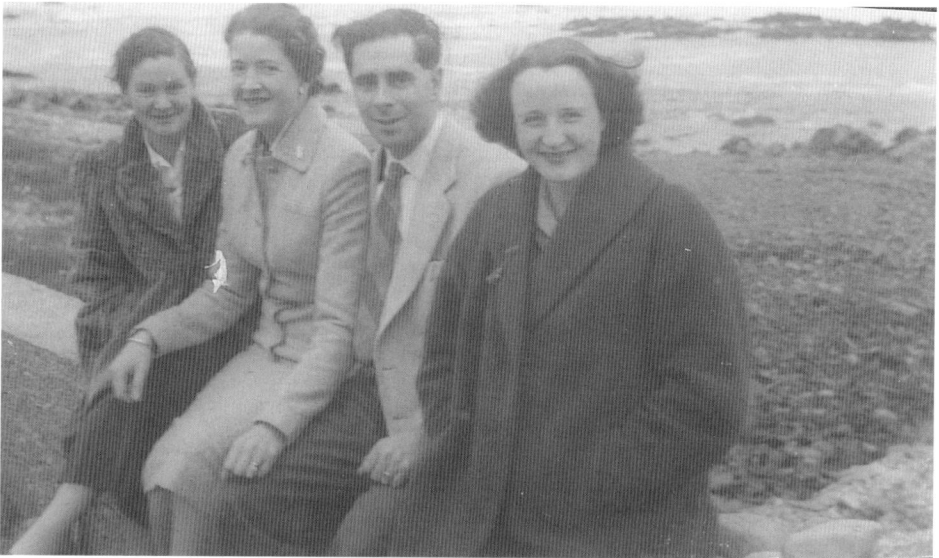

Eileen Corbet, Eileen, Ken and Maura Meade, Malin Head. (Autumn 1957).

1957 –58

Holidays in Cork and Ballyconneely

In June in 1957 Eileen and myself had our first holiday together. By March 1957 we had purchased our first new car, which was the new type two-door Ford Anglia. Eileen was now expecting our first child in August.

We decided to do a trip to our family homes so having installed a locum we drove the three hundred and thirty-six miles from Moville to Castlemartyr in Cork where we stayed with Eileen's family for a week. The weather was beautiful and we enjoyed some wonderful days on Garryvo and Whitegate beaches. We had then toured via Kerry to Ballconneely for a week where we soaked up the sun on Ailbrack and Erriseask beaches before returning through Westport and Sligo to Moville.

The first of our three sons was born at the end of August and in September Adian and Maura who were now back in Dublin came to visit us. I remember that was around the time the Russians put the first sputnik into space.

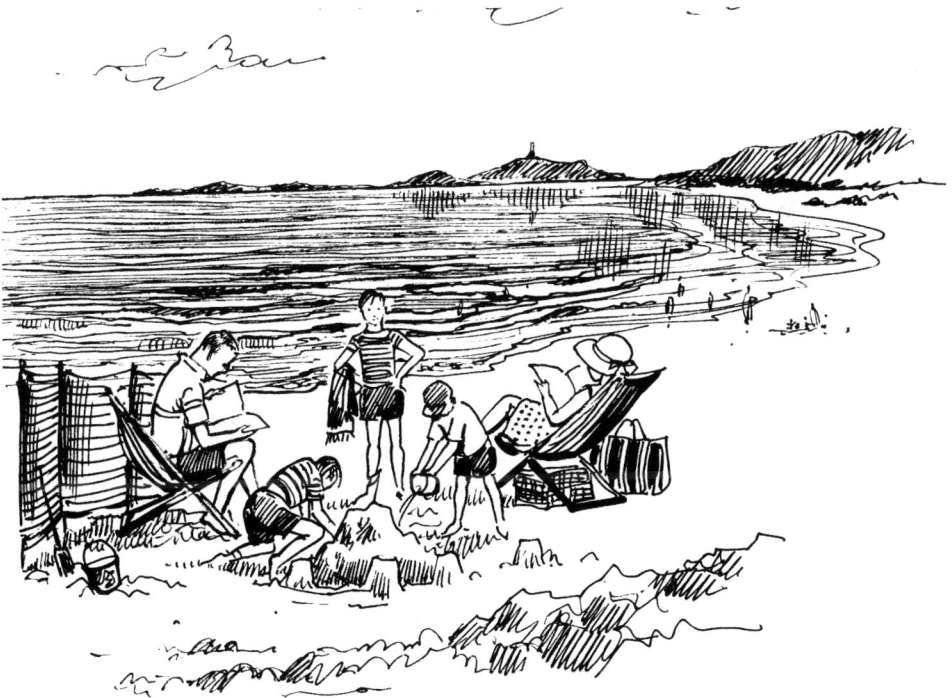

From Slyne Head to Malin Head, A Rural GP Remembers.

The Leaving of Ballyconneely

By now Bernard had taken over Ballyconneely and, as I previously stated, all three of us disliked the pub business. He had now put it up for sale and had carried out a deal with the land commission to exchange the large farm in Ballyconneely for a farm in County Meath. We decided to visit the home in Ballyconneely for the last time so we did this bringing our five-month-old son with us in early January 1958 and stayed for a few days.

Carmel and myself were in full agreement with Bernard's decision but the whole thing would have been very emotional for our parents. The plan was to rent a house near the farm in Meath and build a new house as soon as possible.

As time went on Bernard and his family went back frequently to the Ballyconneely area for holidays. We had one holiday in the hot July of 1972 in Erriseask House Hotel beside the beach where I swam frequently over the years in Ballyconneely. Due to the magnificent weather of that July it had to be the most enjoyable family holiday we ever had.

In January 1958 I came across an ad in the newspaper which appeared to be an unique holiday for Eileen and myself. It was about a trip to Lourdes which began in Cobh by boarding the luxurious trans-Atlantic liner the Mauretania which would be on its way to Le Havre in France, then travelling by train from there to Paris for four days then by train to Lourdes for five days and then returning to Paris three days before flying back to Dublin.

We would normally be going to Castlemartyr which was only a few miles from Cobh so Eileen's mother would drive us there to the tender to board the liner. I was always very impressed by my Aunt Kathleen's description of the liners crossing the Atlantic. Eileen had often stayed with her aunt who lived in Cobh so she was very familiar with the liner traffic coming and going to the port.

I had a very deep conviction that to survive in general practice or any stressful occupation that a good holiday at least every year was essential and that it was planned or arranged several months in advance so that looking forward to it was a great benefit when the 'burn-out candle' began to flicker.

1957-58 was a very busy winter, which had been proceeded by the infamous Asian flu which occurred in August in 1957 and which I had the misfortune to pick up. I got off lightly but I swore that it would never catch me again because at that time the World Health Organisation was developing an anti-flu vaccine, which would be available the following year so Eileen and myself had our forty-fourth anti-flu vaccine in 2001.

In the early summer of 1958 the dispensary doctor in Moville became ill so the council who then was in charge of public health asked me to cover his practice until a new doctor was appointed. I informed them that I would cover two weeks only and that I was going on holidays and that I did not wish to take on the temporary job as the workload would be intolerable and I had no ambition to take on a dispensary job. The double work was a nightmare and I was certainly glad that it only lasted two weeks and that I was then going on our planned holiday.

Paris Holidays 1958

Having left a locum in charge we drove to Cork and were driven to Cobh by Eileen's mother and got on board the Mauretania, which was waiting.

We were thrilled with exploring our way around the decks and the big lounges and dining rooms and we certainly enjoyed the voyage to Le Harve and vowed that we would cruise again. We were thrilled in Paris viewing the famous buildings and shows. The overnight train trip to Lourdes was a great experience and we enjoyed the few days there and the return train journey back to Paris. We then flew back to Dublin and took the train back to Cork and after a day of rest returned to Moville.

On arriving home we found a different doctor installed in the house who quickly explained that he was the dispensary locum and that our locum had left either for personal reasons or more likely from pressure of the workload. The council again asked me to take on the temporary job but I informed them that if I was immediately appointed permanent and pensionable at the age of sixty and with reasonable off-time arrangements I would consider it. Needless to say my demands were not acceptable but they did employ a succession of temporary doctors until 1960 when a permanent appointment was made and this was Dr Jack Magnier, a Corkman, who became my colleague and friend for over thirty years.

New Arrivals

In the fifties and later when a mother was in labour or giving birth the husband took a back seat and while he may have been around he was barred, by convention, from attending and witnessing labour and delivery. I was and still am inclined to agree with that convention. In my case with the workload that I had it would be impossible.

When our second son was born in 1959 I was extremely busy and obtaining very little sleep and the night before he was born I was involved with a prolonged and difficult labour and delivery and was up all night and that night I drove Eileen to the nursing home in Derry. When she was installed there I went home and collapsed into bed. During the night the phone rang and I managed to lift it to hear Sam, the obstetrician, talking and presumably informing me about the details and outcome of her labour. Relieved that I did not have to get up on a call I immediately fell into another deep sleep and when I eventually woke up I had a very vague idea that Sam had been on but I had no idea of what he said or was I dreaming! After a short time I decided to ring the nursing home and 'Bluff' when the matron answered I said 'How are things?' she replied 'Great your wife and the little boy are sleeping' if she had said baby instead of boy I would have been no wiser. So I got it in one.

I am sure that would have been the situation with many GPs when their wives were delivering with phones and doors always ringing. I often wondered how we ever managed to achieve pregnancies! However our third child was born in 1961 presumably during the day and that completed our family.

The Sixties

By the early sixties I had completed over five years in General Practice and I felt that I had a sound knowledge of the area and the people. On looking back the sixties stick out in my memories, as being the toughest of the three and a half decades of my working life, parts of it were nightmares and other parts very exciting.

As the fifties drew to a close the scourge of TB was slowly coming to an end with the great work of public health doctors and the arrival of streptomycin. Polio was still around and I had the sad experience of attending one adult patient who had the virulent type and sadly died in hospital.

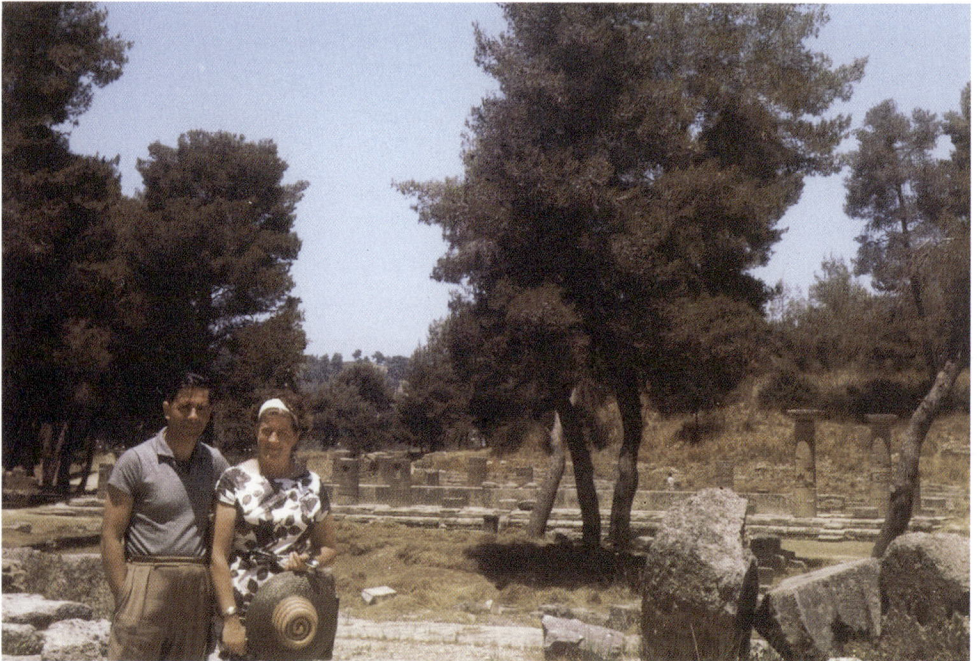

Ken and Eileen, at the ruins of the stadium where the original Olympic games were held in Greece. (1960's).

The Flu

Huge flu epidemics seemed to occur every winter and this led to extremes of workloads. The elderly were the big problem as they all appeared to have chronic bronchitis probably due to the whole population smoking, this caused infection and acute bronchitis which then put pressure on the heart which in turn brought on acute congestive heart failure when the lungs filled up with fluid and this invariably occurred at night between 2 and 4 am when the patient was lying flat in bed. This always led to a very genuine night call for the doctor and clergy.

In those days we had only one real heart drug and that was digitalis, which was originally made from foxgloves and discovered many years ago. There was also another drug, which was helpful, and this was Amynophylline, which was in liquid form and could only be administrated by injecting into a vein and helped the lungs to cope. The most important procedure was to get the patient propped up to a sitting position in the bed.

The drug required to change all this distress for everybody was a real diuretic (a drug to bring an immediate passing of urine to drain the excess fluid from the lungs). There was a drug 'Mersalyl' which was of little benefit and very poorly tolerated. The real diuretic was to come in a short time and this was Lasix or Frusemide, which changed the whole scene.

It was available in tablet and injection forms and tolerated by everybody. From the GP's point of view it has to be the most dramatic breakthrough since insulin and antibiotics and certainly guaranteed many more restful nights for GPs and clergy.

Confusion and dementia was another problem in elderly patients with flu usually occurring at night when the patient got out of bed and wandered around the house and going out during the night to tend farm animals. This caused considerable stress to the relatives and extra night calls for the GP. The problem would eventually clear up when the chest infection cleared.

These flu epidemics in the sixties were real nightmares for me doing up to twenty plus calls per day over a vast area and in the pre Lasix days twice daily to give an Amynophylline injection and in some cases a third during the night. While examining a patient in one house messages were coming in to attend next-door neighbours and this went on and on. I frequently fell asleep in the car and on occasions I pulled into the roadside for a sleep and on waking up I had no idea where I was or whether I was coming from or going to a particular call and had to refer to my diary to check if the call had been crossed off. Frequently I drove up wrong by-roads. On arrival home I would often slump over the steering wheel and fall asleep.

There were times when I got out of the car to go into our house I would look across the Foyle where the lights of Magilligan Prison in Northern Ireland would be shining brightly I almost envied the inmates who were now presumably sleeping.

During all this mayhem there was the occasional call to a trawler or a big ship at the Foyle Buoy, or a drunken driver in the Garda station to carry out a 'section forty niner'. This was the examination of a drunken driver long before the blood test system had arrived. On many occasions the drunk could stand up much better than I could! There were also frequent calls to maternity cases (this was the time to book the extra holiday to the sun well in advance to occupy my mind during the height of an epidemic).

In order to reduce the flu epidemic workloads I went to extreme lengths to persuade as many elderly people as possible to take the anti-flu vaccine every autumn. The amount of vaccine supplied by the health board was a joke so I did a deal every year with a drug rep to get a large supply of vaccine at cost price. I had no interest in charging a fee as reducing the epidemic even by a small fraction was worth much more to me.

Snow and ice was another problem which could complicate flu epidemics. Fortunately they did not always coincide but when this occurred it reduced the number of calls but it took much longer to do the reduced number so I was back in square one.

Snow

Due to the hilly terrain in Inishowen snow was a problem, which I hated intensely and vowed that I would never go on a skiing holiday. When called out during snowy weather people gave as much assistance as possible where there was deep snow on hills. The cars in the sixties were much better for driving in snow than the more modern cars, which are almost useless in the conditions.

I used the big Ford Consuls while they were available in that era when I did an average of 36,000 miles per year and changed them every two years. In those years of frequent snow it was the custom in this area to fit 'weather master' tyres on the drive wheels during the winter months. These were big tyres with large grips similar to jeeps and they certainly helped in any sort of moderate snowfalls and could climb hills if there was no drifting.

The use of special chains was another system, which was really a crude method (as they were used only when required and the car had to be jacked up to fit them on the two drive wheels a most unpleasant experience on the side of a hill on a freezing night). Eventually a more satisfactory system came from Scandinavia, which were clamps that could be fitted on the two tyres in four minutes.

In addition to all the above systems for battling against the snow loading the boot with heavy objects like concrete, blocks, bags of sand, large stones and the most important equipment a spade and an ash shovel.

The Man in the Boot

On one memorable occasion I was helped by two brothers (farmers) who were doing their utmost to push the car and myself on that last effort to the summit of a long steep hill. As we were not making progress we reckoned that another bit of weight in the boot could help to bring success so I asked Sam the shorter of the two to sit in the boot on top of the blocks and stones and away we went to the top of the hill to reach the level road. Sam told that story to many people for many years and reminded me of it every time we met. It is such memories that make it worthwhile!

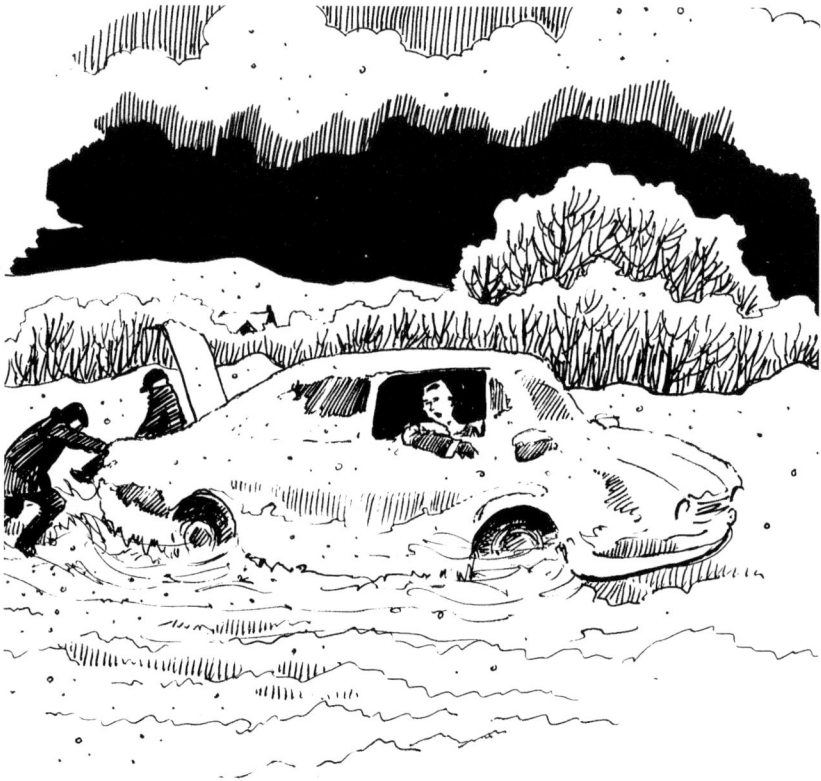

From Slyne Head to Malin Head, A Rural GP Remembers.

The Consul in the Snow

I remember one night Eileen and myself had a meal in the City Hotel (long since gone) in Derry and then went across the street to see a film in the cinema (also gone).
It was a very cold night and there were occasional snowflakes around. When we came out of the hotel the place was covered in deep snow so we had to dig all around the Consul to get it moving and eventually out of the city and on the road to Moville. It was that very fine type of snow and as it was fresh it was possible to drive but as we progressed drifts appeared.

As we pressed on we found that we were ploughing through the drifts with the snow coming up over the bonnet and across the wind screen so we were hoping against hope that we met nothing but hopes were dashed when about two miles from Moville we met a van being pushed up a hill outside a pub so we had to slow down to get around it. Having lost momentum we came to a halt in the middle of the road on a hill.

As we sat helpless and discussed and dismissed the possibility of walking the rest of the journey, a large lorry load of flour came along so the driver and helper both of whom we knew well came to our assistance. They cleared away the snow from the wheels and placed jute bags on the ground in front and behind each back wheel. We then got moving for the final push home.

Early the following morning I got a call to a house in Iskaheen back along the same road and then up a steep hill. When I got the call I was reassured that a farmer would supply transport on a tractor for the climbing part of the journey. There were frequent trips on tractors when it was impossible to drive a car off the main road. On all these occasions the people concerned or their neighbours were always very helpful and gave directions where to meet.

The tractors in those days were not as comfortable as the modern machines and had no passenger seat in the cab. I was made as comfortable as possible with a few bales of hay or straw in the link box in the back of the tractor.

I had a hair-raising experience when travelling in a link box in a small open tractor when descending a steep hill on an icy road with the tractor slithering from side to side.

I had the awful dilemma of deciding to jump onto a ditch or stay put as both options were dangerous I decided to stay put and hope it would not turn over. Eventually the driver got it into a shallow ditch and all was well.

On another memorable occasion when I had a white Consul with a black sort off plastic roof and I was visiting two houses half a mile apart the road had a covering of frozen snow so I drove very slowly on the narrow road to the second house and when I arrived at the door the lady of the house greeted me by inquiring if I was taking my cat on my rounds. The pussy had got on board the roof at the previous house to get the heat I have no doubt that she returned home safely.

During all the years I had only one serious accident on snow and ice and that occurred when I thought I was driving very carefully on a gritted road in a six months old BMW. There was snow and black ice on the road and while going very slowly down a hill and much to my horror the car suddenly went into a skid across the road, hit a wall and crossed to the other side up a ditch and hitting a telegraph pole and capsizing on its side on the road. Apart from the shock I had no injury due to having a seat belt on. The big worry was the possibility of a large truck or any vehicle approaching would skid into the car so I got out very fast to warn approaching traffic.

In a very short time several vans and cars had arrived and everybody was anxious to help and in a very short time got the car back on its wheels and towed to the garage where I was given a loan of a car until the BMW was repaired.

Death in the Snow

This is the final episode of my experiences in the snows of the Donegal winters and certainly the one I remember vividly. This was a sudden very heavy fall of snow around 8th December in the late sixties. I got a call in the morning to a house about six or seven miles away and as this journey was on the main road with little or no hills I felt I could get there with the aid of chains on the wheels.

My two older sons were off school so I brought them with me and all went well until about a mile from our destination where the snow got deeper and the chains appeared to be of no great help until the car suddenly came to a halt. We all got out to investigate and found that the chains had pushed the car so well that the snow had built up under the car until it became impacted and lifted the body off the road so that the wheels just spun around.

We were on a long, straight, flat road. There were no houses and no visible help to be seen so we got down to work I with a spade and the two lads with ash shovels until we had cleared the impacted snow and went on our way to our destination.

On the return journey near Moville we picked up a young man walking in the deep snow on his way to the town.to get a doctor to go to a glen, known as Glenagivney, where an elderly man had collapsed and died while attending his sheep in the snow. He had certainly got lucky! The system in these circumstances was that doctor notified the local coroner who would then instruct him to examine the body and report back.

Where this death occurred is a beautiful scenic area made up of four glens; Glenagiveney, the Long Glen, the Mossy Glen and the Far Glen. All four glens meet north east of Inishowen Head sweeping down to the beautiful and historic Kinnego Bay and facing out to the North Atlantic, Scotland and the Isles.

Like many beautiful places glens can become very hostile environments in snowstorms and gales and this 8th of December was no exception and being one of the shortest days of the year was no help.

There are now three roads into the these glens so after a rushed lunch I drove a few miles to board a tractor at the beginning of the road into the Long Glen. Snow was falling and darkness was rapidly enveloping the short evening as we progressed slowly to reach Glenagiveny and the residence of the deceased.

Having carried out the required examination I had to wait for a long time for a large tractor with a cab, which was conveying the coffin, the undertaker, his assistant, a

Garda and a relative of the deceased.

By the time the undertakers had finished their work the snow was still falling, darkness had long since descended and a wind had come up. Despite these conditions it was decided that all five of us would make a bolt for it on the tractor. I was given the place of honour beside the driver in the cab along with the guard. The other two had rigged up a discarded table, upside down, on the buck rake of the tractor. This whole set up would have appeared as 'Scott's' last trip to the Antarctic.

We decided to take a route with the corkscrew hill, which descends several sharp bends over Kinnego Bay.

As we reached the hill to descend there was a gale blowing down from Scotland forming a minor blizzard.

As I had a good knowledge of that stretch of road I got my head out of the cab to guide the driver. With the aid of a scarf over my mouth and nose I could manage to breath. This was the scariest experience I ever had in snow and I was certainly relieved when we reached the level and straight road.

The only problem then was to stay on the road as on some stretches there were no walls, ditches or hedges to guide us but the 'back seat drivers' on the upturned table on the buck rake could just see the tips of rushes appearing occasionally over the snow and shouted directions to the cab. When we reached the main road the men hooked my car to the tractor and towed me to Moville to bring to an end that December day and night which is etched in my memory.

Whenever I meet the driver during severe snow conditions we always recall that journey in the glen down the hairpin bends.

The Therapeutic Drug Era

During the sixties and onwards-new therapeutic drugs began to appear for the treatment of various illnesses and conditions. This development made life much easier for the GP. In my experience the arrival of Lasix (Frusemide) was a giant leap forward for the treatment and relief of congestive heart failure and made life much more tolerable for the patient and GP and also helped to prolong life for many people.

Cortisone could be classed as the greatest discovery despite its side effects in its early days. More refined forms are still used in acute allergies, asthma, organ transplants and arthritis.

New drugs such as Ventolin also came on the scene to replace adrenaline and ephedrine. In the treatment of asthma other more effective drugs and various types of inhalers and nebulizers replaced steam inhalation and the historic 'potter's asthma cure' which was inhaling fumes from an herb on a saucer.

I remember seeing elderly men in Jervis Street sneaking to the toilets with their matches to 'set up' this potter's cure when the adrenaline and ephedrine had failed to give relief.

There are numerous heart and blood pressure drugs being replaced by new discoveries almost by the week. Advances in psychiatric and chemotherapeutic treatments are forging ahead. The old chronic gastric and duodenal ulcers are now well controlled by new drugs such as Tagomet and several successors so that gastric surgery is now rarely required.

There is now such a profusion of drugs that it could be difficult to see the wood for the trees but we are still much better off than the days when we had very few drugs and less technology.

I felt privileged as one who has experienced the relatively hard times and appreciated moving into the good times with the benefits of the rapid advances of pharmaceutical research and medical technology. In my time while extremely busy in surgeries my obsession with not rushing may have been a good thing. I remember when a drug rep called he or she had no appointment and neither had the patients filling the waiting room but they had no problem in directing the rep into the surgery when the door opened. I always found these visits very relaxing while discussing the latest drug and then moving on to discussing the All Ireland Finals or the most recent rugby or soccer international. Meanwhile in the waiting room the patients were all relaxed and discussing the weather.

Planting the Roots

In 1962 we purchased the rented house from the elderly landlady who owned it. From the start we had been very happy there and the landlady had kept up replacing lost slates and repairing any structural damage but would not permit us to carry out any internal structural change and she did not wish to sell either but in May 1962 she did offer to sell so we bought it immediately without any haggling.

So after seven years and three children in Moville we now had the roots firmly planted so we could undertake any structural changes that we wished. Our first priority was a new roof followed by numerous other changes and developments over the next five years.

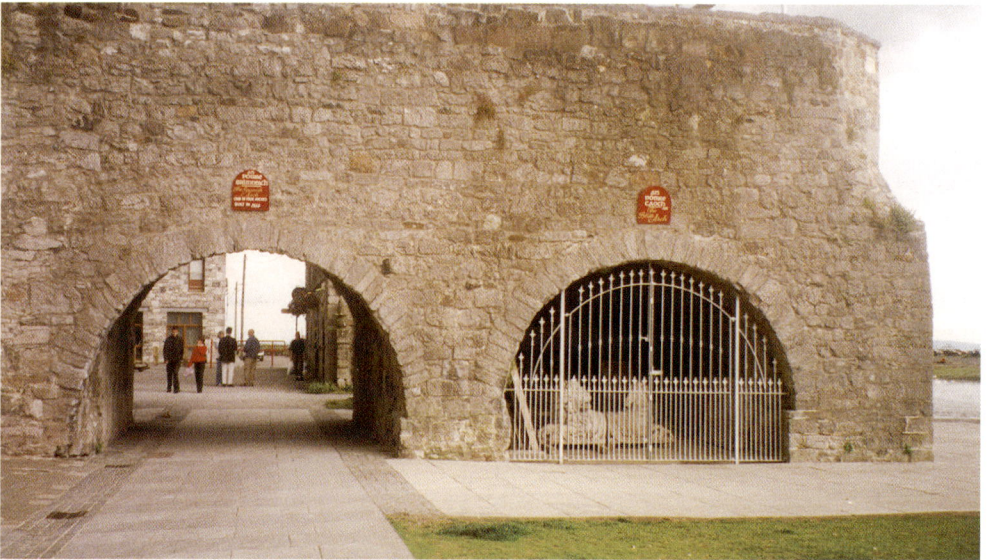

The Spanish Arch, the Claddagh, Galway.

Hurricane Debbie

Many strange things occurred in the sixties and one was Hurricane Debbie that hit Ireland on 16th September 1961 causing havoc over the country. Eileen and myself had gone to Dublin on the previous day to attend a wedding on the following day. The ceremony was in Donnybrook Church and the reception in Portmarnock Hotel. Before and during the ceremony when a door opened flowers and altar decorations were blown around the place.

On the way across the city to Potmarnock we could feel the strength of the wind rocking the car and Dublin Bay was in a frenzy. While in the hotel during the day we were oblivious of the havoc going on outside. Those were the days when weddings were held in the morning and the reception ended in the late afternoon.

When we left for home and heard the news on the car radio we were horrified at the reports of the widespread damage and the vast number of trees blown down causing mayhem on all roads and widespread damage to buildings, stripping slates and tiles off numerous dwellings. We concluded that our chances of reaching Moville that night were nil. However we pressed on hoping for the best and after several miles we were amazed how well the roads were made passable despite the number of fallen trees. Considering the small amount of heavy machinery that was available at that time the council workers and others certainly did magnificent work in clearing a passage through the fallen trees to allow traffic to proceed so we were encouraged to keep going.

Somewhere on the Monaghan side of Castleblaney our progress was slowed down by me developing a dose of diarrhoea, which forced many stops, which included climbing over the fallen trees and opening gates to do what I had to do! Despite my predicament we kept going until we reached Redcastle only four miles from home. This was a very wooded area so that a very large number of trees had fallen probably late in the day so that the road was completely blocked.

My knowledge of the back roads then came to the rescue as I hoped that taking a connecting by-road over 'Croc-a-naina' a high hill in mountain land and bog where there were no trees so I could connect with another main road to Moville. The gamble worked so we eventually reached home, as I was about to 'stagger' into bed there was a loud knock on the door requesting me to visit a lady well on in pregnancy. She was suffering from shock due to a large tree falling on her home fourteen miles from Moville.

Due to the very unusual circumstances I had no difficulty in driving the distance to see her. The men who come with the message had cleared a passage on a narrow by-road at Redcastle so it was possible to drive directly to the call. Fortunately the patient had no complications and eventually had a normal delivery around the expected date.

Deaths in the Family and Dallas

On the 19th November 1963 my father died as a result of a stroke, which came on suddenly a week earlier. He was then aged 74 years and living with Bernard's family in Killmessan Co Meath. The funeral on 21st went from Killmessan on the long journey to Ardbear cemetery on the Ballyconneely side of Clifden. My cousin Fr Bernard Lee who died suddenly from a heart attack the following week performed the graveside ceremony. His brother Michael had died the previous March.

We stayed in Clifden on the night of the 22nd and headed for Moville on the following day. It was a rather sombre trip and we did not have the radio on but somewhere along the road between Ballintra and Laghey approaching Donegal Town we decided to turn on the 6 pm news and that was when we first heard of the shooting of John F Kennedy in Dallas Texas.

Rossapenna

The sixties were full of surprises and rare experiences. From our early days in Moville despite the hard work we tried to explore the beautiful countryside of northwest Donegal. During the summer months we would try to escape from the work on a Wednesday, which was our 'official' half-day.

So to get to the neighbouring Fanad peninsula and the area around Mulroy Bay it was necessary to drive the forty miles to Letterkenny to get started. On our anniversary, the 14th June, we would go for a meal in Rathmullan House situated on the beautiful western shore of Lough Swilly. On some occasions we went to Carrigart or Rossapenna on Mulroy Bay and drive around the famous Atlantic Drive and have a meal in Rossapenna Hotel.

This was an old establishment, which was built on the Scandinavian or Swiss styles with a huge amount of wood used in its construction. It was built on a golf course, which was a great amenity for attracting tourists. We had celebrated our anniversary there on a few occasions when the weather would be living up to the month of June. It was a wonderful trip on the rare endless days of June in north-west Donegal.

In May 1961 the priest who married us was on holiday with his mother in Donegal and they were staying in Rossapenna Hotel so they invited us to have dinner with them in the hotel. We enjoyed the pleasant journey and were looking forward to meeting our friends.

As we drove in the road through the golf links to the hotel I remarked to Eileen that it appeared somewhat odd that I could not see the hotel where it should be seen. She replied that I was probably looking in the wrong direction!

At that stage I remembered seeing smoke over a hillock and when I reported this to Eileen she replied are you telling me that the hotel is on fire or what?

We then saw our friends in their car waiting for us on the road and then we both saw the heap of smouldering ashes that remained after the hotel had burnt down to the ground in half an hour. Fortunately, or miraculously, all the residents and casual visitors were at lunch in the dinning room on the ground floor when the fire started, so everybody including staff and visitors escaped without injury.

The hotel guests were accommodated in the near by Carrigart Hotel and we had our meal there. Eventually a new Rossapenna Hotel was built on an adjacent site.

Disaster on Belleighan Hill

In the early sixties there were R.A.F. bases in Eglintion and Ballykelly on the eastern shores of Lough Foyle. At one stage in those years a large aircraft flew out at dawn to bring weather reports from the north Atlantic. There were also small combat or training planes which frequently could be heard flying over the Foyle north of Inishowen Head. At that time these were normal sounds audible most days.

On one foggy, miserable November day the sounds appeared to be very loud, vibrating and very close to Moville but not visible due to the fog. I remember this experience very vividly as at that time I was walking into the local post office where the staff and customers were speculating as to what was happening. Just as I arrived home for lunch there was a phone call from the local vet on his two-way radio to go to Belleighan Hill where two R.A.F planes had crashed.

This area was approximately four miles north of Moville towards Inishowen Head. Eileen and myself went off realising very well that our meagre supply of emergency equipment would go nowhere on this job. On arrival at the scene we found that two small aircraft had flown straight into the side of the hill situated a few hundred yards from a dwelling where an elderly lady, her daughter and two sons resided.

The air was thick with the smell of aviation fuel and there was burning wreckage scattered over a wide area. There were either two or three partially charred bodies in the wreckage of each plane.

On viewing the scene two things struck me the first was the vast amount of small parts like nuts, screws, bolts and numerous other bits and pieces scattered over a wide area. The second was trying to imagine what the sight of a large civil aircraft with over a hundred passengers would be like after a crash.

As far as I can remember British and Irish military personnel arrived as we were leaving to attend the shattered family where our main function was to try and counsel the elderly lady and her daughter and given them some sedation which was very much required after their horrifying experience.

The Doctor Patient
and the Sick Doctor

Doctors like everybody else are human and can develop a drink problem like anybody else due to having easy access to drugs for relieve of pain or any psychiatric problems he or she can try to treat himself or herself instead of consulting another doctor.

In order to address this problem there is a scheme within the medical fraternity known as the sick doctor's scheme.

This is a group of doctors who volunteer to give advice and counselling to those with problems and to persuade them to consult another doctor or specialist for help before it's too late.

In March 1963 probably due to exhaustion, cold weather and bronchitis I developed pneumonia and was compelled to take time off. I had great difficulty in obtaining a locum but eventually succeeded and a bright, middle-aged man arrived in the late evening and was very keen to start work and get on with some house calls that were in the town.

Eileen went with him to give directions but before he got started he went into a nearby pub for a brief period and then proceeded to do the calls. When he returned he produced a bottle of whiskey and got to work on it! It was originally arranged that he would stay in the house as we had plenty of space. On going to bed he had difficulty in climbing the stairs. Eileen was shattered after this brief experience and my first reaction was to tell him to leave but on second thoughts we decided to leave it until the morning and when asked to go he got up and left.

This was the pathetic and sad case of man who was once a brilliant young doctor. I then asked my colleague Jack to cover for me until I recovered. I was delighted to return the compliment when he had pneumonia some years later.

Hooked on Joyce

As far back as the mid thirties I had often heard my parents referring to a Dr. Oliver St John Gogerty who had a hotel in Renvyle, a well known tourist seaside resort, where he also had a residence. The area was around ten miles from Clifden and near the mouth of Killary Harbour, Ireland's only real fiord. He was a throat surgeon and his wife was a Duane from a nearby townland and her brother Matt Duane used to stable his racehorses in our stables in Ballyconneely on the eve of the Errismore Races.

The memory of those references to Dr. St John Gogarty and the association of the horses and Errismore Races remained very much in my mind and when Ulick O Connor published the biography of Gogarty in 1964 I was very anxious to read it. I had two good reasons for this the first was to learn more about Gogarty and the second was because Ulick O'Connor was a contemporary of mine in U.C.D. He studied law. I did not know him personally but he was a well recognised all round athletic and successful in boxing, pole vaulting and rugby. No doubt this endeared him to Gogarty who was also a brilliant athlete in cycling and swimming.

In the mid sixties I had no time what-so-ever to read a book apart from medical journals and during holidays I spent most of the time sleeping. Probably in May or early June in 1965 I purchased a hardback copy of the book. I could not resist reading it, so on a warm Whit Monday Bank Holiday, when I was supposed to be off, I went to the magnificent Culdaff beach and hid, curled up on a warm sand dune, with skylarks flying higher still and higher overhead, I read the whole book by literally scanning and flicking the pages and stopping here and there to read a few paragraphs. Gogarty fascinated me but I was also very struck by the many references to Joyce and his friendship with Gogarty, albeit a short one, but became immortalized in Ulysses. Prior to this my only knowledge of Joyce was that he was a man from Dublin who wrote banned books. I was now 'hooked' on Joyce and there will be more anon.

Portstewart and Portrush

During the summer from around the mid sixties until 1969 we frequently took the three boys to Barry's amusements in Portrush on a Wednesday afternoon providing that there were no maternity calls or other emergencies. Being 'off' on Wednesday afternoon frequently involved several repeat house calls between Moville and Muff before completing the fifty-six mile journey to Portrush (this was twenty years before the Foyle Bridge was erected).

This journey included driving through Derry and crossing Craigavon Bridge to the eastern side of the Foyle and proceeding northwards, parallel to the Foyle and Inishowen, passing through Limavady, Coleraine and Portstewart to reach Portrush and on to the roundabouts, swings, bumper cars, slides etc. Barry's was a large establishment on a permanent site and is still there and the next generation is about to move in.

When it came to the chicken and chips time I would phone home to inquire of the housekeeper if there were any urgent or maternity calls and if so we returned home, if not we had our meal in Portstewart and then returned home.

Very frequently on our return there would be calls with or without one or more patients waiting in the waiting room that was the way it was.

I had a four to six hour break and if I had to work for part of the night so be it but things were about to change.

The trips to Portrush ended in 1969 when the real troubles started in Derry. In the winter months of the sixties we occasionally took the boys shopping in Derry and then had a meal in the Melville Hotel then where the Foyleside shopping centre is now located. We all enjoyed the Melville on cold winter evenings. It had a large dinning room with a lush red carpet and a blazing fire. We enjoyed the meals there and if we got lucky and got no calls we went to the pictures.

Breakthrough in Technology

At some stage in the sixties my colleague Jack Magnier led the way in modern technology when he obtained a telephone answering machine. I had never heard of such a machine but I was informed at a later date that the A.I. station (artificial insemination) had one for some time. After discussions with Jack I also got a machine installed.

These were not purchased but rented, which included service and just as well because these machines frequently broke down. These original machines were huge compared to the modern micro machines. These machines were as large and as heavy as a television set and contained masses of wires and two large reels resembling cinema projection reels with similar tapes, which frequently snapped but could be easily repaired with sellotape.

For all other repairs the renter had to phone head office in Belfast to send a technician who frequently had to take the whole machine to Belfast for repairs.

With all its problems it was without doubt a great help particularly to the spouse of the GP who no longer had to answer the phone every time it rang.

In addition to answering the incoming calls the early machines could relay messages to the owner when away from home. The owner activated this operation by using a code system. By the use of shouting in sharp words or digits for e.g. ONE-ONE-ONE etc four times then after a brief cracking sound the tape would reply the recording of any messages received. In the early days of the machine the recording could include bad language using colourful expletives. I had an amusing incident when calling the machine from a phone box in the Errigal Hotel in Letterkenny. As I was using the code to activate the relaying of messages there was some confusion by two men discussing buying farm gates. I was not sure if one was in the box next to me but the other certainly was not, my code was confusing them and they were certainly confusing me. As I was repeating the code the farmers were becoming more confused and frustrated so we were all shouting the farmers shouting at each other and shouting at my machine eventually one of them shouted 'what the hell is all this one-one about?' At this stage I gave up and made the call later.

As time went on the machines were being replaced by smaller and much more efficient models which could be purchased directly at much lower cost until we are now in a completely different world with minute mobile phones, e-mails, web sites etc. What I write today will be history in a few weeks.

The End of the Sixties

As the decade moved on, and the renovation and the structural changes to our house were eventually completed, we began to think of the future and decided that another house, on a good sized site, would be a very secure investment for retirement if we survived long enough and in the meantime it would be there for relaxation when regular off time would eventually come which was inevitable. We asked a builder to look out for a site I felt that having come from the land that I had a desire to own a small amount so I could enjoy gardening. I was always a passionate believer in having a retirement and the earlier the better. Not by any stretch of the imagination could I see myself working over the age of sixty-five.

As Jack and myself were almost living beside one another we began to realise that there was no sense of both of us being on call at weekends when one could easily cover the same area and despite the fact that dispensary doctors had no weekend arrangements in their contract by this stage was ludicrous. We decided in 1968 to jump the gun and do alternate weekends. We then arranged real weekends from 4 pm on Friday to 8 am on Monday. Like Neil Armstrong on the moon it was a tiny step but a giant leap forward into the twentieth century.

Around 1970 a county physician who was president of the medical union succeeded in obtaining official weekends off for dispensary doctors this was a short time before the G.M.S. came in.

Around Easter around 1969 we got the site which was slightly over an acre and which was situated over looking the Foyle between Moville and Greencastle.
We decided to build in about two years and in the meantime we were very happy with the sense of security and with the alternate weekends off. We could look forward to developing a garden.

School and Death

In September 1969 the eldest of our three sons went to Castleknock. Between the three being there, with two years between each starting, their time was spread over ten years which happened to be the first ten years of the troubles. They usually travelled by bus from Derry to Dublin and now that I had alternate weekends off we had no problem visiting them on a free weekend.

At that time, in 1969, my mother was ill from lung cancer and she had been with us in Moville from September 1969 to February 1970 when she returned to Kilmessan and sadly died in May at sixty-eight years of age and was buried with my father in Ardbear cemetery in Clifden. Tragically like many others she had paid the price of smoking but at least her generation did not know of the danger.

The Seventies

THE SPANISH ARMADA AND LA TRINIDAD VALENCERA

In 1588 King Philip of Spain or (Philipus Rex in Spanish) and Portugal decided to invade England. He organised a large amount of ships to form a fleet known as The Armada to sail to England and carry out the invasion.

This armada consisted of one hundred and thirty ships made up of warships and converted large merchant ships many of which were confiscated from their owners. This fleet carried thousands of soldiers in addition to the crews and at that time would have been the largest force of warships ever seen.

They sailed for England in the summer of 1588 but when they reached the English Channel they were routed by the British fleet and forced to sail up the east coast of England, around the north of Scotland, then across the north Irish coast and down the west coast of Ireland where many of the ships were wrecked in storms. It was recorded that one of the ships 'La Trinidad Valencera' was wrecked in Kinnego Bay in northwest Inishowen in the parish of Moville. This is a beautiful horseshoe shaped beach and a very popular place for bathing and picnics during the summer months.

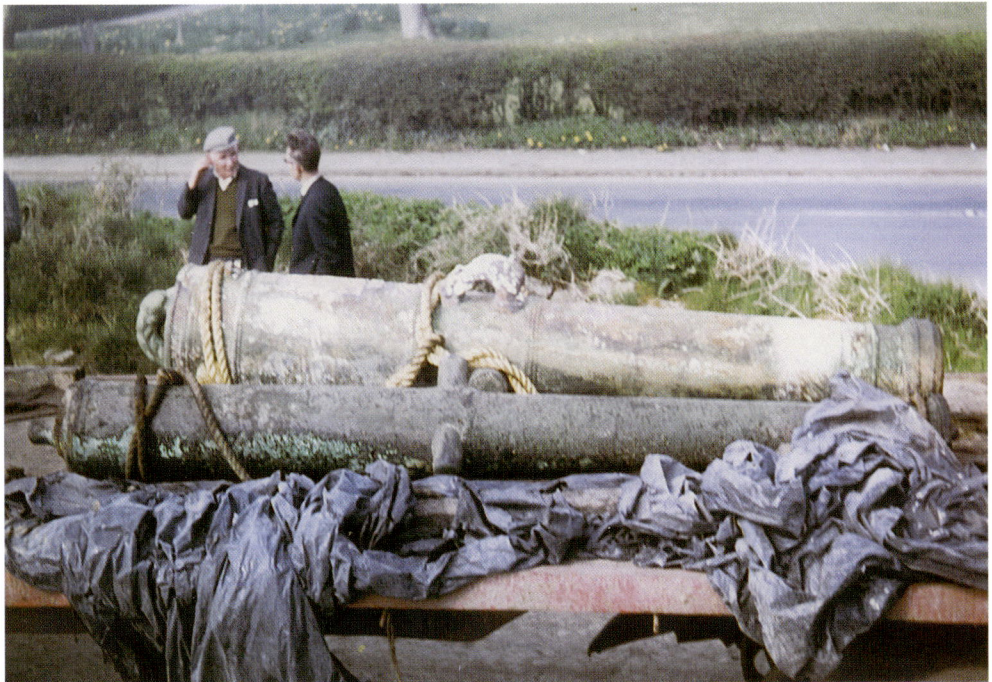

Spanish Armada Cannon.(1972)

From Slyne Head to Malin Head, A Rural GP Remembers.

When our family were young and I had weekends off we frequently had picnics there and we usually sat on flat rocks, which jutted out into the sea for about two hundred yards close to where the 'La Trinidad Valencera' was lying for almost four hundred years.

The wreck was discovered on a cold February afternoon by the Derry Sub Aqua Club when one of its members noticed a circular object protruding from the sand and from closer inspection found that it was a thick metal circular object and possibly the barrel of a large gun. All the divers there searched the area and discovered more objects probably more guns so they were satisfied that they had discovered the wreck of 'La Trinidad Valencera'.

The club then decided to keep a low profile and notify experts to carry out a scientific marine archaeological excavation. They then contacted Colin Martin of St Andrew's University who at that particular time was carrying out a series about Armada wrecks on BBC 2 and he agreed to act as archaeological director so the excavations began a short time later in April.

It was Easter so I was off for the weekend and the boys were off school. We were all extremely interested and excited about this great discovery and we were very fortunate to almost have 'ringside' seats and glorious weather to witness the raising of one of the large guns from the sea bed onto a trawler. We just wallowed in watching these massive ancient guns being winched up out of the sea only a few yards away and to really put the icing on the cake I got a photograph of the large gun just as it was being winched out of the sea, three hundred and eighty three years and seven months after sinking in Kinnego Bay on the 16th September 1588. The guns were transported by trawler around Inishowen Head to Carrickarory pier in Moville and then hoisted onto an open lorry where they were officially photographed on this Easter Sunday morning. I climbed up on the lorry to get my own historic photographs.

The excavations went on for a long time and a huge amount of artefacts including coins, footwear, plates etc were discovered and are now in the Ulster museum in Belfast. The large gun is now in The National Museum in Dublin.

During the excavations, which were carried out during the summer months the archaeologists, had a tent erected on the shore and they had temporary accommodation in a vacant house nearby with a sign over the door reading 'La Trinidad Valencera'. The following is taken from a plaque on a pedestal erected high over Kinnego Bay at the entrance to the road leading down to the beach

The Spanish Armada

Here in Kinnego bay on September the 16th 1588 the merchant ship the 'La Trinidad Valencera' of the Spanish Armada broke her back and fell apart.

La Trinidad Valancera was a Venetian merchant ship pressed into service with the Levantine Squadron if the Spanish Armada.

At one thousand one hundred tonnes she was one of the largest ships of the fleet and carried forty-two guns and some three hundred and sixty men, two hundred and eighty one of whom were soldiers.

About forty lives were lost when she sank and some three hundred and fifty survivors including those from other ships reached the shore. More than two hundred of these were killed outside Derry by a force under Rickard and Henry Henendon.

The City of Derry Sub-aqua club discovered the wreck of the La Trinidad Valencera in 1971.

This plaque, which commemorates the four hundredth anniversary of the Armada, was erected by Bord Failte, Donegal/ Letrim/ Sligo Regional Tourism Organisation and Donegal County Council in 1988.

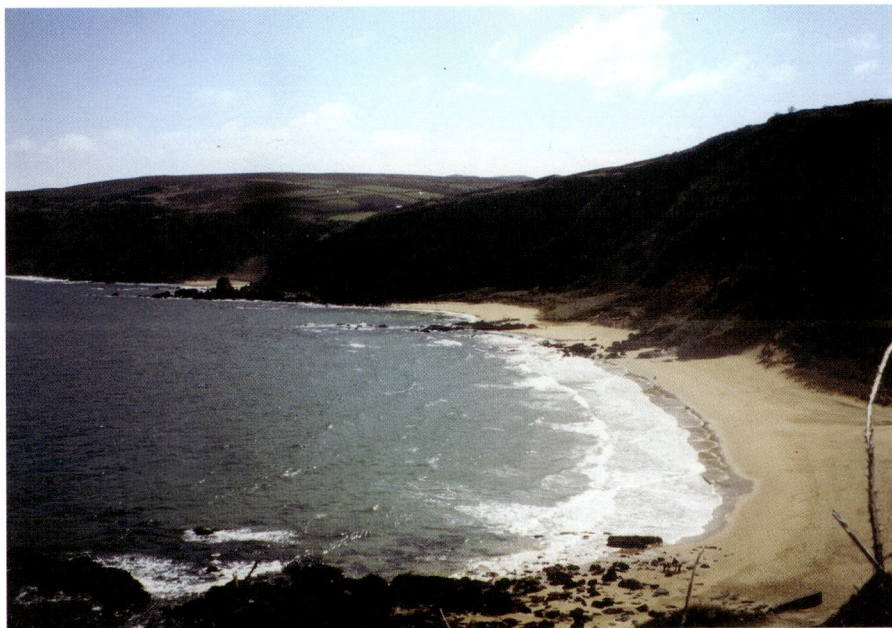

Kinnego Bay

From Slyne Head to Malin Head, A Rural GP Remembers.

Ballybrack

As mentioned previously, we had decided not to build for some time but later we were advised to go ahead as soon as possible as building would become more expensive when Ireland would join the EEC as it was then called.

In January 1972, the Wednesday before Bloody Sunday, we asked our friend and neighbour, Liam McCormick, to draw up the plans and apply for planning permission and asked a local builder to undertake the building which began in July 1972 and was completed in March 1973. We now had security for retirement and in addition enough ground for developing a garden and as I now had alternate weekends off I was about to enjoy it.

We then developed a routine on these weekends to travel the one point seven miles from James Street Moville to Ballybrack. The weekend was from 4 pm Friday until 8 am Monday. I had resolved from the beginning not to take homework with me and with my colleague on duty there was no question of seeing patients there.

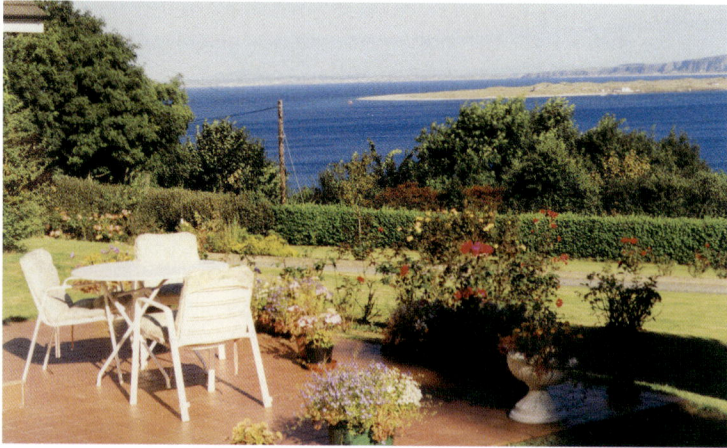

Above:
View from Ken's
home, Ballybrack.

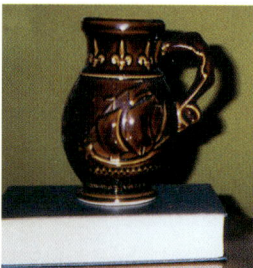

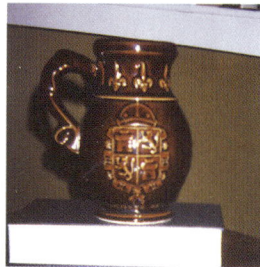

Left: Rear view of tankard from a commemorative set celebrating the discovery of the Trinidad la Valencera in Kinnego bay in 1972
Right: Front view of the tankard.

The New General Medical Service

(The GMS)

As was inevitable the dispensary system was slowly drawing to an end to be replaced by the new general medical service. Negotiations and plans had been going on for years until eventually it was agreed that the new system was to be called the GMS was to begin on 1st April 1972 and was phased in by first starting in the Eastern Health Board on 1st April 1972 and the rest of the health boards on 1st October 1972.

This general medical service was also referred to as the 'choice of doctor scheme' which was one of the big differences with the old dispensary system where one doctor was appointed to a district so that the eligible patients could only attend that one doctor, where as in the new scheme patients could have a choice of doctor.

When the scheme started any private doctor who had been at least five years in the area could join the scheme and take on eligible patients.

The payment of doctors was changed from a salary to a fee per item of service, which involved a large amount of paper work for keeping records of doctor's claims and fees. On the day the new scheme started on 1st October 1972 I was exactly seventeen years in practice in Moville so I had no problem in joining the new system. I remember registering my first patient in the GMS, which was a house call at 12:15 am on 1st October 1972.

With the increase in paperwork I had decided to employ a full time practice nurse as I was convinced that it would be impossible to run a practice without efficient professional assistance in the surgery. I was certain that another doctor as partner or assistant was not the answer as while easing the amount of outside calls, paperwork, and filing records would become chaotic the answer to that problem was waiting in the wings.

This was a nurse Greta Rawdon who was living with her family in the town. She did her training in the Mater Hospital in Belfast where she worked for some time as a theatre sister. After working in various positions she was appointed district nurse in the Moville area where she worked for ten years and during all that time she was a working colleague of mine so she had the perfect experience as a practice nurse. So when I asked her she was delighted to accept the position and I was certainly thrilled at the prospect of working with a nurse with her experience and wonderful personality. After three months notice to her previous employers, The Local Nursing Association, she began her work as a practice nurse on 1st March 1973. This was a great and thrilling day for both of us to quote Yeats

'Everything changed,
Changed utterly'.

I had been waiting for this day for seventeen years and now that it had arrived and that I had fulltime professional help in my surgery and alternate weekends off, when I could relax and enjoy the garden, I felt that the seventeen years wait was worth all the hard work and sleepless nights.

By coincidence I was into the second half of my career as a GP and I was hoping that with a good slice of luck I would reach an early and satisfying retirement.

Doctor in the Air

For many years Eileen and myself were very 'slow learners' in gaining confidence in air travel so with some trepidation in the summer of 1974 we decided that the whole family would fly to Lourdes on a package that had a week in Sans Sebastian and three days in Lourdes.

We had frequently heard of passengers becoming ill during flights and the cabin staff calling for a doctor to attend an ill passenger. Up to this time I always considered myself too ill from fear to get out of the seat and walk to the sick passengers. Invariably (that is until this time) another doctor would volunteer.

Around half way through this flight to Lourdes a call went out for a doctor and I fell asleep until I got the elbow in the ribs from Eileen and then the three lads in front turned around saying 'go on dad'. So after another brutal nudge of the elbow I got out of the seat and the Holy Ghost immediately descended on me and brought the power back to my legs and that was the last I saw of my family until well into the night I then swaggered along the aisle up to the front seat where the patient was seated.

This was a lady who had a small degree of heart failure and was obviously distressed but not in any real danger. The cabin crew had supplied oxygen and supplied me with a stethoscope. The patient had her supply of medication so at this stage all I could do was frequently check her pulse and keep her reassured.

An air hostess did not reassure me when she whispered into my ear that there was torrential rain and thunderstorms all around Lourdes and the Pyrenees and that conditions in Lourdes were so bad that the flight would probably be directed to another airport but they were not informing the passengers just yet.

She also requested me to remain with the patient and accompany her to the hospital when they landed and that the airline would arrange transport to the hotel for the rest of the family. Things were now becoming dramatic but the real drama started when we did land directly in Lourdes in the torrential rain where the patient and myself were transferred to a small ambulance with what I first thought was a 'mad' driver, screeching around the town at one hundred miles per hour which reminded me of the famous trip in the Coombe ambulance. Fortunately it suddenly dawned on me that I was reading kilometres instead of miles on the speedometer. I was relieved to known that the speed was actually over sixty miles per hour in the rain. Having left the patient in the hospital I had a joy ride to the hotel.

Years later there was another call for a doctor on a long haul flight but being now ten years retired I felt very satisfied in allowing a 'real' doctor to take charge.

The Sick Doctor No: 2

Around June 1975 despite having alternate weekends off and time to relax at my gardening and the great help and assistance from my practice nurse I began to feel very tired with a great loss of energy I was convinced it was not a recurrence of the TB as I had no sweating but I kept hoping that it would go away. Unfortunately the symptoms persisted so that when I finished surgery in the afternoons I headed for our new house in Ballybrack and having set an alarm clock I would take a deep sleep for an hour. At that time one of our sons was learning to drive and was about to do the test so when I was doing calls I got him to drive while I slept in the car while doing house visits. This crazy setup went on to the end of July when I had a long weekend off on the August Bank Holiday and I looked forward to having a long rest. When Tuesday morning came I could not contemplate getting up for work and for the first time I had a temperature and a slight cough.

To complicate everything my colleague Jack fractured a leg and had it in a big plaster cast so that he was off work but fortunately he had got a good locum who was a very good young doctor and agreed to cover my practice as well as Jack's until I could get a locum.

After having x-rays and various tests the conclusion was that I had virus pneumonia, which would require several weeks rest. I was very much relieved to learn that I had nothing worse and did not require any special treatment apart from rest and above all I could now lie in bed all day and sleep despite the fact that there was glorious weather outside. At this stage the locum was working away in the two practices and would visit me every night and one night he looked me straight in the eye and said 'it is no wonder you are lying there exhausted from over work'.

He had been called to one of my patients several miles away and when he arrived there the patient's wife informed him that he wanted to have his blood pressure checked when the locum inquired where he was at that time she said that he was in a byre looking after a sick cow. The locum was horrified at this and rightly felt that this was an unnecessary call and that many of these patients could attend the surgery.

I fully agreed and was delighted that he had brought up the subject because I had been considering this for a long time and I knew I was 'on a roundabout' and finding it very difficult to get off. This set me thinking and I rapidly concluded that I now had the perfect opportunity to jump or putting it another way I had already fallen off so I made a definite decision to change the system immediately I returned to work so the embryo off the first co-op was formed.

In the meantime I had been trying to get another locum and I was relieved when one arrived but not all that happy because he appeared to be over age for a locum but he appeared to be very enthusiastic and was very anxious to stay on and become an assistant. At that stage I was clutching at straws and considering the proposition.

Meanwhile 'back on the ranch' in the surgery Greta was having problems keeping things going as the locum was creating considerable confusion. Eileen and herself did not wish to worry me but when it came to a crisis point I was informed we had another sick doctor on our hands which we had to let go very rapidly and notify the health board. Fortunately Jack's locum was still available but could only remain until the end

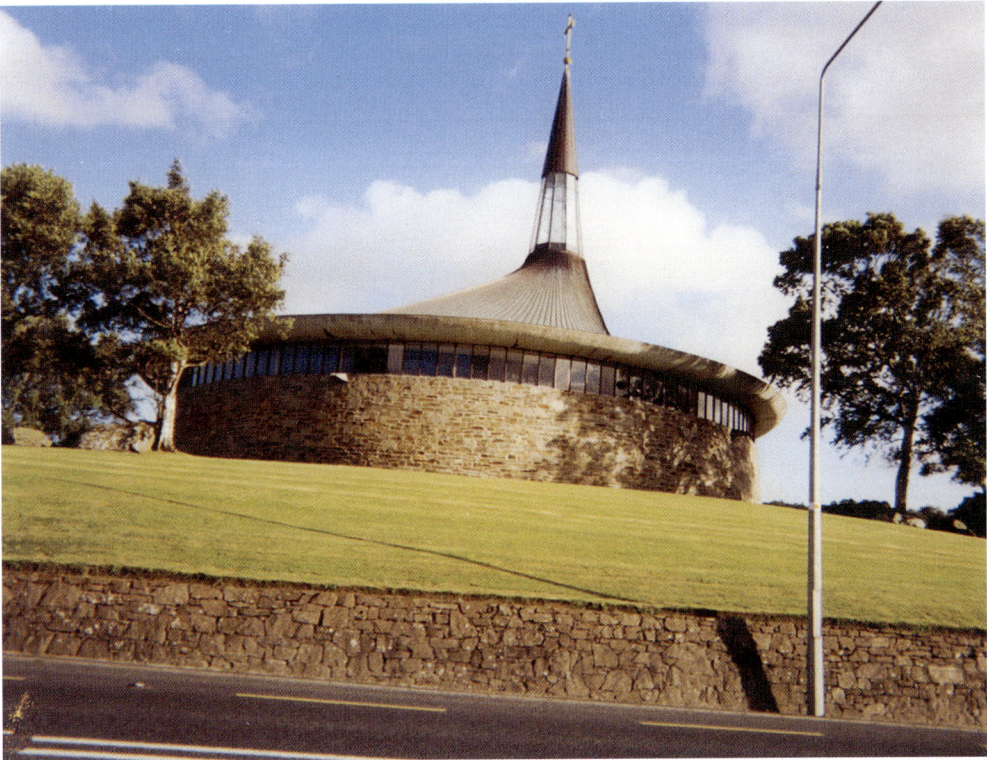

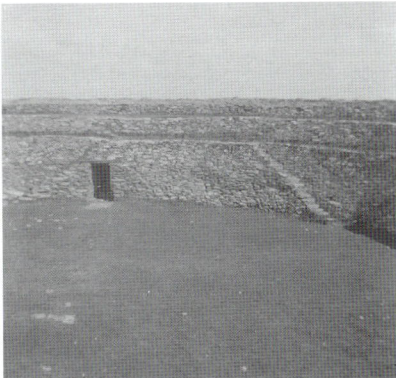

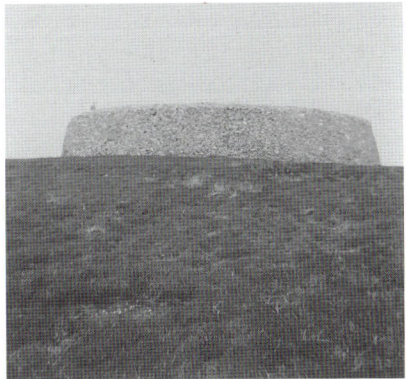

Grianan of Aileach

of August so I set about obtaining another and had better luck this time around. This was a young, confident man who remained for several weeks and who was interested in staying on as an assistant or partner and agreed to work with me for a few weeks before I returned to full time work. He was engaged to be married and had no problem living near Northern Ireland in the height of the troubles as it was at that time but his fiancée was horrified at the idea and would not come near the place. So that was the end of that and I then decided to put the idea of assistant or partner out of my mind, put the head down and go for it. I had Greta in the surgery and Jack around the corner so with continuing co-operation we had reasonable off time.

I remember a colleague living near the border once saying that it was extremely difficult to persuade a locum to come north of Mullingar not to mention coming near the border.

In my observations, Galway graduates had no problem going into Northern Ireland to do training in northern hospitals and later working in border areas in Donegal.

After making a full recovery and Jack's leg not fully recovered we had a discussion that now was the time to change the system and persuade patients to make more use of the surgery instead of unnecessary domiciliary calls.

As the patients appeared to be glad that both of us were back they were anxious to co-operate so we changed the whole system around in a short period.

I frequently made the point that when I came to the Moville the only cars in the parish were a few hackney cars, the priest's car, the clergyman's and the doctor's but in 1975, twenty years later the priest, clergyman and the doctor still had one car each but most households had a least one or two cars so by then it was easy to get transport to convey many adults and all children to the surgery.

This arrangement made the system more efficient by reducing the amount of time driving large mileage around the country so that more patients could be seen at the surgery.

The Troubles

Living thirteen miles from the border most people lived with the proximity of the mayhem that was going on in the north from 1969 until 1994. Despite frequent bombing of pubs and business establishments, blowing up bridges and shooting of individuals, life, business and transport went on as near to usual as possible. Tension was sporadic and would be more noticeable at times during bombing or marching events.

We went in and out of Derry frequently and just lived with the checkpoints. The customs had always been on the border so that remained normal but a short distance away on the northern side there was a large army checkpoint where there was the installation of a large tower, ramps and obstacles slowing down cars and other vehicles. During all these years in going to Derry it was necessary to allow time for possible tailbacks of cars and trucks.

The usual routine was for a soldier to request the driver to let down the window and he would request to see the driver's licence or other form of ID and usually requested the driver to open the boot. On some occasions the driver would be asked where he or she was going.

The vast majority of people had no problem with this and if they had they kept it to themselves. There were always the occasional drivers who delayed everything by questioning the legality of the various requests of the soldier and this futile attitude made the delays worse and built more hassle for the individual himself or herself on future crossings as the security had the registration number of all cars so they would recognise belligerent drivers very easily.

My personal attitude on all occasions was to get through as soon as possible so I never had a problem except once when a bag of 0-10-20 fertiliser got torn in the boot of my car a short time previously. This alerted a sniffer dog and then I remembered to explain to the soldier who just had a close look inside the boot and waved me on.

There were also several checkpoints around the city to check pedestrians where the routine was similar to airports. On some occasions there would be a bomb scare so that a street or part of a street would be cordoned off. All this became routine and people walked the streets and did their shopping as usual.

When there were contentious marches or threatened riots it was advisable to avoid the city as the shops would be closed and your car could be hi-jacked and ruined but life would return to normal the next day.

Our three sons travelled by bus from Derry to Dublin to boarding school so between secondary school and college there was almost always at least one travelling on that route over a span of twenty years of the troubles. During the boarding school period Eileen and myself drove frequently to visit them.

On the journey to Dublin there was a very large checkpoint at Aughnacloy where there was the same routine as the one near Muff and on very many occasions on dark and late winter nights we checked in and out without any problems through both checkpoints.

We did have one 'hairy' incident, which was not a checkpoint. We occasionally visited friends in Monaghan on our return journey from Dublin and one night we left there around 11:30 pm.

Somewhere between Newtownstewart and Strabane we got boxed into a convoy of army trucks and other military vehicles. This was a very frequent occurrence either day or night in those days. This was a rough night with lashing rain and high winds. There were two soldiers with guns at the ready sitting in the back of the truck ahead of us. When we reached Strabane and going towards Lifford Bridge the convoy halted.

As we sat there facing the two guns at around 1 am it was lashing rain and there was a big sheet of corrugated iron banging on an old gate. There were tin boxes and cardboard boxes being blown around. The whole scene reminded me of a post war film I saw around 1950 called Harry Lime played by Orsen Wells.

As my thoughts returned to the scene in the back of the truck I remember saying to Eileen what we do not need now is somebody throwing a petrol bomb, she replied, 'could you not think of anything more cheerful?' I replied that I was only joking but she was not amused.

After about fifteen minutes, which seemed much longer to us the convoy moved on and eventually went on another road so we got on our way to Moville in one piece.

Another experience occurred during the time when streakers were fashionable in public. Around that time drivers were requested to go into a hut at some checkpoints and sign a book. This really got up the nose of the perpetual objectors. On one occasion I was asked to sign so I said certainly 'I will sign anything except a blank cheque'. As I was signing an officer in the hut said, 'We're looking for you'. I knew immediately that he was joking I replied 'what did I do wrong?' He replied 'you were seen streaking in Dungannon yesterday', my reply was 'you can be bloody sure I wasn't streaking in this lousy weather'. He replied, 'I would agree'. As he said 'Cheers' I returned to the car.

In the summer of 1969 I remember witnessing a part of confrontation between the police and residents in the Bogside when stones and CS gas were being exchanged. On one occasion when going through the city to meet one of our sons at the bus I was held up by a policeman who informed me that there was a bomb about to go off some distance ahead and that there was a warning of another bomb some distance behind so for about half an hour I felt like a mouse in a barrel, driving up and down various side streets to get out but they were all obstructed in various ways. Eventually I got to the bus stop and got home via some diversions.

There was one occasion when I could have been in the wrong place at the wrong time. For some years there was an open car park at the bus terminal and while waiting to meet the incoming Dublin bus I would walk up and down the length of the car park to get an extra bit of exercise instead of sitting in the car.

On this occasion, on an Easter weekend, I was off duty so one of our sons drove to Derry to meet one of his brothers. He had a friend with him and while waiting in the car a bomb went off very close to them. It caused no damage to the car but the explosion sent out a flame along the ground that got very close. The explosion killed the bomber. If I had been meeting the bus I would have been out walking and could have been in the wrong place at the wrong time.

On another occasion I got a call to a house near Muff, which was situated some distance from the main road, and a narrow road went along by the border to this house. A helicopter frequently patrolled this area. I was not familiar with the road so I was driving very slowly and I noticed a helicopter flying closely overhead. It had a very strong searchlight and became almost stationary when I stopped to go into the house and when I came out and got into the car it moved off.

One Christmas Eve morning Eileen sent me off to Derry to get some last minute Christmas shopping that had been forgotten. On the return journey near a petrol station on the Derry side of the border I saw a large lorry reversed in half way over the kerb and there was a few men around, one of them was holding what I thought was a big spanner in his hand. He waved me down to stop so I obeyed the instruction.

After a few minutes he came to the window holding the spanner but it was not a spanner it was a revolver or handgun definitely a gun of some description. He informed me that it was now OK to move on. I learned later from the media that an ambush was being set up. This was my one and only direct encounter with a paramilitary operation.

The Scalp

In all rural areas GPs did a considerable amount of casualty work particularly in suturing (stitching) of all sizes and descriptions providing there was no damage to tendons or nerves and that excess bleeding could be stemmed. It was important to clean the wound no matter how long it would take and to use local anaesthetic.

My great ally for cleaning wounds was what my mother used at all times when we were children and come running to her with bleeding knees, fingers or whatever, this was hydrogen peroxide, one of its properties was to bubble up like a pint when applied to a wound or infection. Another well-known property was useful for changing brunettes to blondes. The bubbling peroxide bubbled out grit and dirt without causing burning like iodine. It was also claimed to have a mild antiseptic property.

I had no ambition to be a general surgeon but I had a great admiration for their skills and their huge responsibility for their patients. I loved minor surgery of stitching and removing benign cysts I could never resist removing sebaceous cysts the bigger the better and the practice nurse was always a great help. I remember one experience that sticks in my memory not so much about the actual treatment but the circumstances surrounding it.

On a summer Saturday night some time in the sixties the surgery was full of all sorts of minor complaints and injuries mostly due to the influx of visitors. In those days I had a night surgery (later abolished).

Around 11 pm an elderly man was brought in with a head wound caused by falling into a shallow river and bashing his head on a sharp stone. When I examined his head I found to my horror that he had been almost completely scalped so that it was possible to lift the scalp from his forehead and peel it back so it could nearly hang down to his neck. There was sand and gravel all over the place as there was very little blood loss at that time I told him to wait until I got the rest of the patients cleared. He did not wish to wait around for a long time so his minder took him for a long walk on that balmy bright night along the shore path. I eventually got to work on him around 1 am and with the help of his minder I spent the rest of the night hours and the dawn cleaning out the sand and gravel with the peroxide and inserting thirty stitches and eventually finished at 7:30 am.

I instructed him to stay in bed for the rest of the day and that I would visit him to check if there were any signs of brain damage or fractured skull. When I got there on Sunday afternoon he was out walking around. The wound healed very satisfactorily and there were no long-term complications.

Sea Angling

The seventies brought in a very exciting and a different memorable phase in our lives. The family were in their secondary school and college phases of their youth and enjoying sport to the full.

The sea angling festival, which started in 1957, was still going strong and our sons were enjoying the excitement in addition to the football, when I had a weekend off during the festival I enjoyed a day out. Eileen's brother Tony was a keen sea angler in Cork and came on a few occasions for the weekend and once for a whole week. With alternate weekends off I would be free to join the fun for at least one weekend. In those days when it went on for two weeks there were several fringe events including shore fishing, a fancy dress ball, street frolics and bonny baby contests.

As time moved on the festival became smaller due to the trawlers becoming larger and not suitable for angling so availability of boats became a problem.

The festival still exists but it is reduced to two weekends while Greencastle has become a very large fishing port.

In recent years an oyster festival has been flourishing in the month of September and this could be classed as complementary to the sea angling rather than competing with it.

Horse Races

When I came to Moville the local races had been in abeyance for some years but were revived in 1973 by a very enthusiastic committee who invited me to act as official medical officer on the racecourse. The meetings were held on the Sunday of the bank holiday weekend and brought back memories of the Clifden and Errismore races. I enjoyed carrying out this pleasant duty every year until my retirement in 1990.

On this duty there was very rarely any work to be done and on the very rare occasions when a young jockey fell off a horse the last thing they needed was a doctor near them as they were always embarrassed and did not wish to admit to any injury so they got up and away as soon as possible. Professional jockeys have no problem when they fall it is part of the job. The Moville races have again gone into abeyance mainly due to the high cost of insurance.

The Running Doctor

In the late seventies and early eighties a movement grew up in the U.S.A. and other parts of the world to counteract the rapid declining of physical fitness. This was due to the rapid increase of motorcars and machinery in addition to huge advances in technology so that walking and manual work were going out of fashion and watching television was a national pastime.

All this led to a decline in physical fitness, unnecessary obesity and heart disease. All this led to a movement in U.S.A. by people taking up various forms of exercise, walking, swimming, cycling, squash and stationary running.

When I recovered from my illness in September 1975 I rapidly put on weight until by January 1976 I was becoming distressed about the lack of my physical fitness. My normal weight of eleven stone had shot up to almost thirteen stone.

I had difficulty in walking up the stairs and even getting out of a car. I had to ease myself out by supporting myself with one hand on the roof. I had a vague recollection of hearing about a jogging movement in the U.S.A. so I began thinking I would have to loose weight.

On one Sunday afternoon in early January 1976 after doing a large round of calls I flopped into a couch and fell asleep and on waking up I suddenly noticed that I had got a large belly and I was about to burst my shirt. I also noticed an opened Observer newspaper which had a large banner headline as follows: 'Middle Age Fitness Time to Act' I was then forty-nine years of age. I grabbed the paper and read rapidly about aerobics and instructions of how to loose weight with little or no stress over sixteen weeks.

The paper quoted from a book written by a doctor in America which was the official exercise programme of the U.S. air force and navy and the Royal Canadian Air Force there were several options of types of exercises for different age groups e.g. from 'stationary running' (also called on-the-spot running), walking, swimming, cycling, squash (before a certain age). I decided on stationary running as it could be carried out anywhere out doors or in the home if necessary in the 'loo'.

This programme for my age in weeks one and two was two and a half minutes stepping up and down seventy to eighty steps per minute counting only when the left foot strikes the floor, on five days per week. When I had finished reading I put on a pair of sneakers, went to the surgery and after the two minutes I had to lie on the couch to recover but I was not seriously stressed. The duration of the exercise very gradually increased until twenty minutes was reached after sixteen weeks.

After the initial exercise I was really thrilled and carried out the rest of the programme on a rubber doormat outside the back door in the Ballybrack house. I was delighted to find I was now only ten and a half stone in weight and I could not believe how fit I had become. Previously I would be exhausted after a few hours work in the garden and had to have a prolonged soak in a hot Radox bath at night to bring some relief to the numerous aches, pains and stiffness.

Over the years I had forgotten what it was like to be fit so I was now determined to maintain it and continued the stationary running six days per week for several years up until 1983 when I changed to real road running during the fun run era.

During that time the fitness cult had become world wide with thousands of people male and female training to take part in the marathons and short distances usually five miles or ten kilometres (6.2 miles) and generally classed as 'fun runs' where athletes could be competing for records and prestige. There would be hundreds running for fun to achieve finishing the race. The idea of the fun runners collecting sponsorship money for deserving charities added to the enthusiasm for the run.

This great phenomenon reached Derry in the early eighties when there were a few five mile or mini marathons confined to women to raise funds for the new Foyle Hospice. On 31st December 1983 there was to be a five mile mini marathon for men. I was beside myself with excitement when this run was announced in the local paper as I knew that after years of stationary running I was certain that I was fit enough to take part provided that I changed immediately to real road running.

I did not wish to run on the public road just yet so I measured the distance from the back door of the Ballybrack house along the gravel path to the gate and back and worked out the distance of twenty-one laps to be three miles so it was easy to convert the stationary running into three miles daily on six days per week. On nearing the fun run it was very easy to very gradually increase the daily run to the required distance. When the day of the mini marathon arrived I was feeling very fit and excited to be back in a public race and with a number on my running vest. For the first time since 1945, thirty eight years previously, in the Iveagh grounds in Crumlin. I ran the race of my life on the cinder track.

There was a difference now in that there was no competitive tension. It was fun and everybody that finished was a winner and had achieved a level of fitness appropriate for their age and would be presented with a medallion.

This first run was from the boat club near the Everglades Hotel on the Strabane Road. It went up the long hill on Victorian Road, then turned left to cross the Foyle on the Craigavon Bridge, then right on the west side of the river passing the Derry walls and the Guildhall to go along the strand to go left onto the Buncrana Road passed St

Columb's College to reach the finish in Templemore Sports Complex. These runs attracted several hundred runners and in the early days spectators lined the streets. An innovation was several real athletes, even world champions, took part in fun runs and were very serious about competing with their colleagues and improving their finishing times or breaking records so this added to the general excitement as the Seiko clock led the run and all runners could check their times as they reached the clock at the finishing line.

From 1983-86 I took part in several runs for charity the most notable was the historic 10 K in early September in 1984 celebrating the opening of the new Foyle Bridge at the northern end of the city in addition to the double deck Craigavon Bridge at the southern end.

The run started approximately half way between the two bridges on the Limavady road on the eastern side of the river and ran down a long hill and a left turn on to the magnificent new Foyle Bridge and across to the western side, then left on to the Strand, the lower deck of Craigavon Bridge, back to the eastern side and Limavady Road to finish at St Columb's Park.

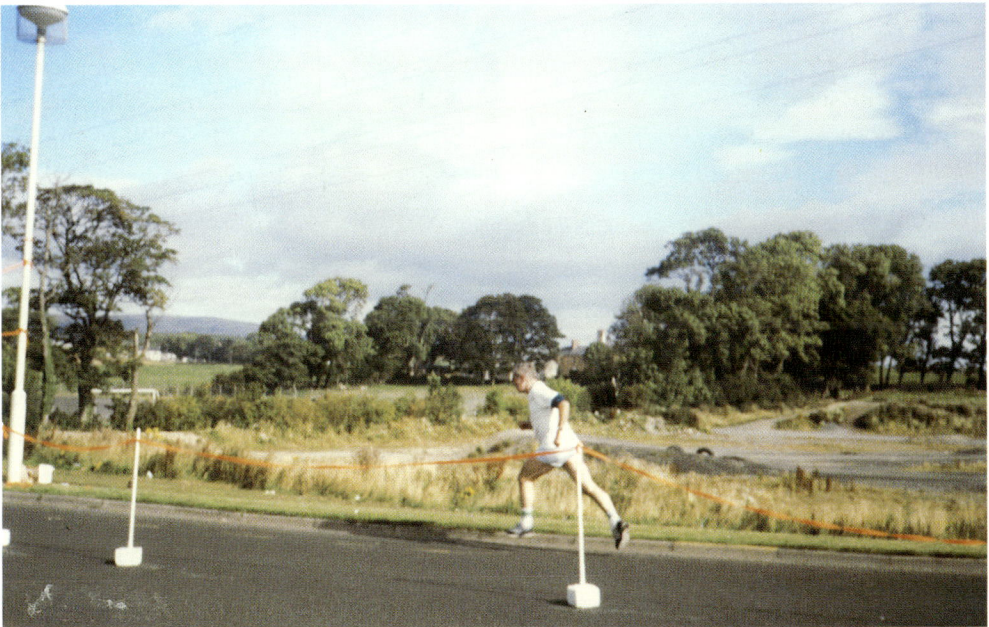

Ken, Mini-Triathlon, Templemore Sports Complex, Derry. (Sep 1986)

Triathlon or Tryathlon

As running was not enough for some enthusiasts. The triathlon was the next challenge and it was not for the faint hearted. This was a triad of events strung together, swimming in the sea or pools, cycling and running. This was very serious stuff and no room for fun runners but not for long.

The tryathlon was invented and this really stirred my imagination and enthusiasm to take on this test. This consisted of swimming ten lengths in a swimming pool (250m), cycling nine miles (15km) and running three miles (5km).

The idea of achieving a tryathlon really thrilled me despite the fact that I could not swim ten lengths of a regular sized pool but like all my generation I used to cycle but I had not been on a bicycle for many years. As I was generally very fit I decided to have a go. After a few trips to the pools in Derry I achieved swimming the ten lengths of the pool at a very slow pace. As Eileen had a bicycle at that time I had to relearn how to ride a bike and succeeded in a short time and was thrilled at renewing my old thrills of cycling. So I was now all set for my tryathlon.

The event was from the pool in Lisanagelvin Sports Complex. It was on a cold and windy September evening and the course was on the outside of the city were there was considerable traffic which made me apprehensive on the cycling leg which was down the hill from Altnagelvin Hospital to Drumahoe and then across to the Limavady Road and the steep climb up the Crescent Link Road to the finish. Just to add to the excitement there was a bomb scare on the way! I got my finishing award appropriate for my age and I was now looking forward to another triathlon. This was the one I love to remember. It took off two weeks later from the large Templemore Complex on a warm sunny morning. This complex was outside the city so there were no traffic problems. The system was that participants went in relays or groups and when the last finishers of each group left the pool the next group started so each individual was timed on leaving the pool. As each swimmer left the pool he or she ran to the changing room and pulled on a T-shirt and running shoes (no waste of time drying) then ran to jump on the bicycle and get away. As my swimming was so poor all the other swimmers of my group had long since gone on their bicycles before I staggered out of the pool to an outburst of cheering and whistling which spurred me on to get on the bicycle where I recovered most of the lost time in the pool as only one of the following group passed me on the cycling leg. The course went along the Buncrana Road crossing the border into Donegal then on to the Letterkenny Road and passed the church of St Aengus in Burt, (modelled on the famous archaeological masterpiece, Grainnan of Aileach,) then a sharp swing to the right on to another road through the famous Burt farm then back to the Buncrana Road to re-cross the border and back to the complex to start the three mile run. When I jumped off the bicycle I fell flat on my face when I started to run but I got up immediately and went on up a hill to a roundabout and back to the complex and the Seiko clock to get the finishers award. These awards were classed as elite, silver, bronze according to time and age of each participant I got the elite award in both trythlons.

For me this personal achievement was a thrilling climax to my efforts to enjoy and maintain personal fitness despite of advancing years when ten years earlier my maximum level of fitness was to achieve two and half minutes of stationary running. This was my second and last trythlon as they became more competitive involving wearing of wet suits and swimming in the sea.

I kept on running 10Ks until 1989 when I reduced exercise to fast walking and tennis but that was not the end the early nineties had yet to come.

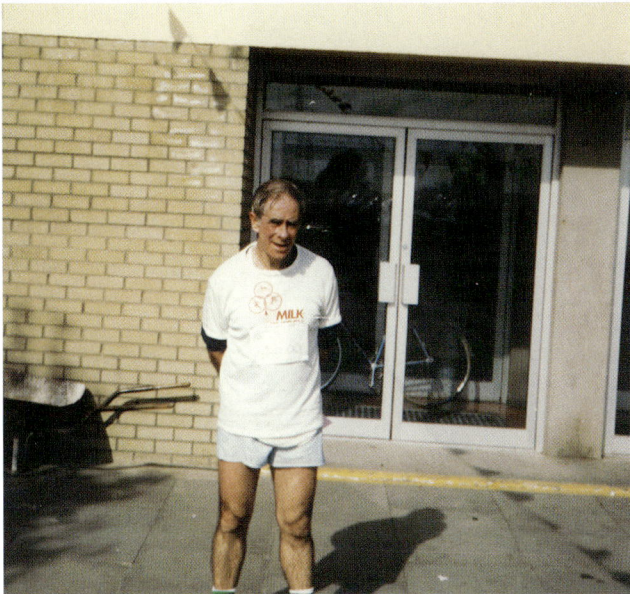

Ken after the finish.

Greencastle

The name Greencastle goes back a long way to the thirteenth or fourteenth century when its Irish name was 'Caislean Nua' translated to English 'New Castle'.

Around that time Richard De- Burgh Earl of Ulster and Connaught built a castle in the area where its towering ruins are still standing. Moville did not exist at that time and was not built until 1820

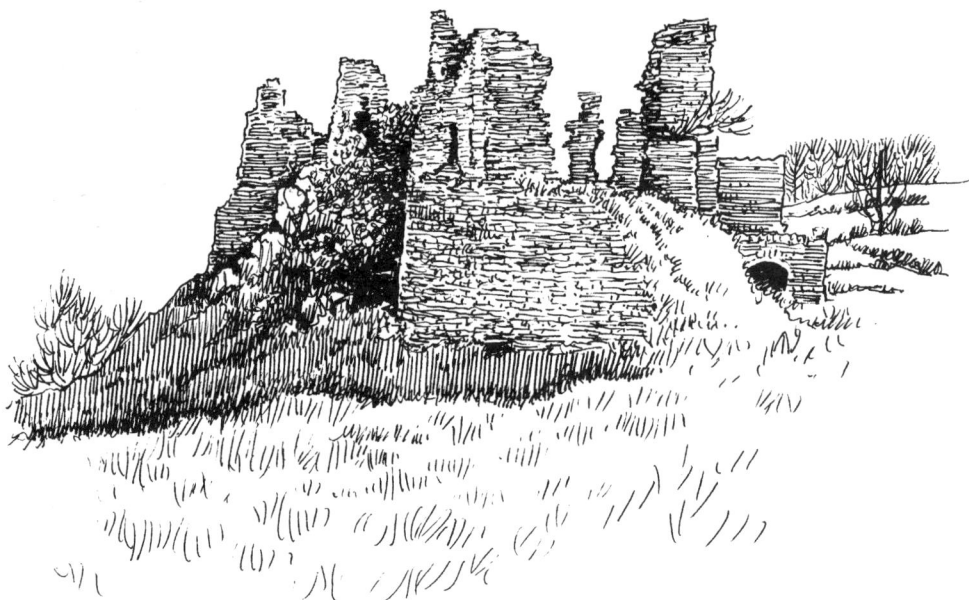

The Fort

In the early nineteenth century there was a threat of an invasion by Napoleon so two Martello towers where built to defend the entrance to Lough Foyle and Derry. One of these towers was in Greencastle and the other across the water at Magilligan Point.

The tower in Greencastle was later to become part of a large fort, which is still standing in its original condition and at present is a thriving hotel and restaurant.

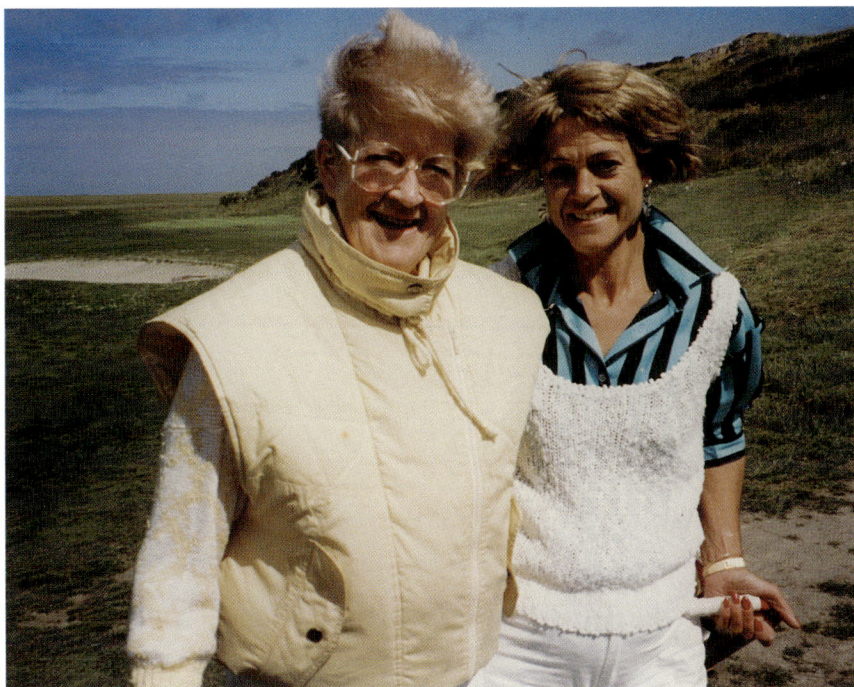

Eileen and Kaye Tighe, golfing partners, Greencastle.

Fishing Port

When I came to Moville in 1955 Greencastle had a small fishing port, which similar to many other areas development was required to keep up with modern large ports and with marine technology.

During the second half of the century huge developments were carried out to deepen and enlarge the port and this was augmented by the building of a national fishery college adjacent to the harbour. The latest development was the building of a car ferry terminal to accommodate a ferry service from Magilligan Point. This has become operational since 2002 and appears to be a great success. The village also has a new planetarium and maritime museum and also a thieving boatyard.

Tragedy

In all coastal areas it is natural for all young men and in modern times, young women to go to sea on merchant ships or trawlers and this occupation has its hazards and Greencastle is no exception.

Over the years there have been tragedies of young men being lost at sea. In November 1995 six Greencastle fishermen were lost when their trawler, the 'Carrickatine', sank off Malin Head. These included a father and son, John and Stephen Kelly from Carndonagh, two young brothers, Jeremy and Conal McKinney from outside Moville and two young men, Terry Doherty and Bernard Gormley from the Greencastle area. President Mary Robinson travelled to attend a Mass and offer condolences in Ballybrack Church. She knew Inishowen very well as she frequently came on holidays with her parents in her youth. This was a sad and tragic time for the whole area and especially for the bereaved families.

Redcastle

Along the Foyle in this part of Inishowen there are two other town lands with the title castle in their names, Whitecastle and Redcastle. I do not have any details of the history of Whitecastle.

Up to the early seventies Redcastle was a large estate which had been in the Cochrane family probably from plantation times. While it did not have a visible ancient castle it had a large manor type house on a large farming estate which was still occupied by members of the Cochrane family and owned by a retired major until his death in the seventies when the whole estate was passed on to a younger member of the family who returned from Canada to take over the house and the estate.

The new owner took over the farm and with his wife opened a restaurant but appeared to have problems clearing debts so the whole estate was sold to become a hotel, which was resold on a few occasions until finally it became a large hotel with a leisure centre, nine hole golf course and tennis court.

The Non-Golfing Doctor

In 1981 my colleague, Jack, and I had agreed to working alternate nights so at long last we had fully entered the twentieth century.

I was now at the peak of fitness playing squash and tennis in the Redcastle facility until dire warnings appeared in the medical journals about the dangers of playing squash over the age of forty so I immediately gave it up and concentrated on tennis which I always enjoyed.

At this stage Eileen decided to take up golf in the new club in Redcastle and that both of us should join and learn the game. I fully agreed and as I now had organised definite time off. I started off with great enthusiasm on the long summer evenings but after two or three weeks I did not look forward to the game and gradually during a game I began to daydream about being back at a packed surgery on a hot, Saturday afternoon with numerous crying and vomiting babies, various accidents causing confusion, anything would be better than searching for a lost ball or waiting around for players ahead to get off a green.

I suffered this overwhelming boredom for the summer while looking forward to the long, dark winter evenings. I was amazed that I had the same feelings at twelve years of age on the old redundant golf course on Ailbrack beach.

Despite all this negativity at playing the game I believe golf is a wonderful game for those who enjoy it I believe that the handicap system is unique in having a level playing field for the average players. I always follow up golf in newspapers and I enjoy watching the big tournaments on TV.

Eileen really loved the game and went on to become Lady Captain in Redcastle for two successive years. She was also a member in the Greencastle Club and played in their winter leagues. She played in the Donegal Alliance League which involved playing in various clubs all over the county. I was delighted and thrilled to know that she enjoyed the game so much.

While she was Lady Captain in Redcastle she received two complimentary tickets from the golfing union for the Irish Open in Portmarnock. We both enjoyed this experience very much despite the fact that it was blowing a gale that day but that did not diminish our enjoyment of seeing the great professionals 'taking on' the elements and Ian Woosnom winning the title.

Smooth Changes 1986

In 1986 Greta retired after thirteen years, which we both enjoyed very much. In the early days of those years she did tremendous work behind the scenes for the development of a day centre for the elderly. This was a great success and had evolved into a much larger and modern centre combined with a large health centre.

She got on with her gardening and enjoying her grandchildren very much for another fifteen years until very sadly after a short illness she died on 2nd May 2001.

Once again I was very fortunate in having a successor to replace Greta. This was Nan McCarron who had a long and varied experience of hospital and district nursing who frequently did relief for Greta so she already had a good experience of GP practice nursing. This changeover was very smooth for patients, Nan and myself.

Jack Magnier also retired in 1986 and was replaced by Dr Don McGinley who had been an assistant in another part of Donegal so he had no problems settling in Moville and being a Galway graduate no problem with the border. He brought with him the technology that was rapidly changing the world – the computer.

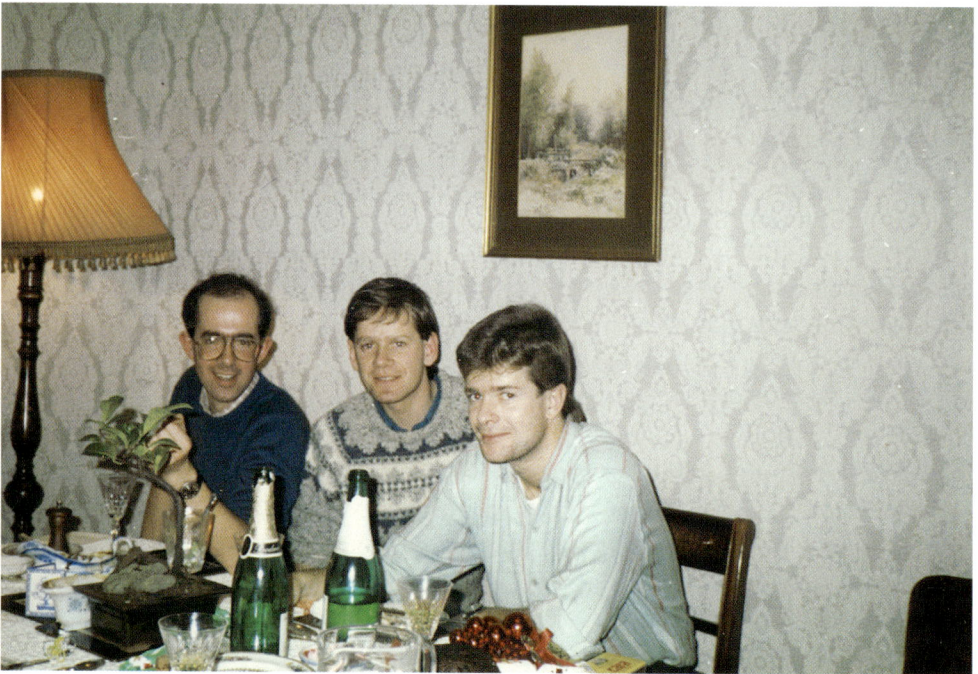

Ken's Sons, Gerard, Ken Jnr and Thomas, Christmas Day. (1986)

The R.C.G.P. and the Birth of The I.C.G.P.

Over a long number of years, doctors in various specialised branches of medicine had formed special groups to keep themselves up to date. There were originally two well known established groups, the Royal College of Surgeons and the Royal College of Physicians founded in the early nineteenth century. In addition there was the Royal Academy of Medicine founded in 1882 this was an umbrella organisation for promoting postgraduate medical education.

It was not until 1950 –52 that the first college of general practitioners was founded and that was in England and was called the Royal College of General Practitioners or R.C.G.P. In order to establish a new college of GP doctors.

All GPs who had least five years of experience where invited to join as founder members and as it developed a special examination would be required for entry into the college.

Irish GPs where allowed to sit this examination and very many Irish GPs availed of this facility until eventually a group of Irish GPs met and formed an Irish college to be known as the I.C.G.P. The new college used the same system as the R.C.G.P of inviting experienced Irish GPs to join as founder members and eventually developed an exam system.

The I.C.G.P was officially born on 29th March 1984 after a long gestation period of several years of very hard work and dedication of a number of GPs led by doctor Michael Boland from Skibbereen Co. Cork. In May 2001 he was installed as president of The World Council of General Practitioners in Durban South Africa

The Oz Experience

Around 1986/89 two of our sons, one a film editor the other a GP, doing the rounds of gaining experience went to Australia to gain more experience and widen their horizons. While they were there, Eileen and myself had been considering paying them a visit and at the same time seeing, at least, a little of that vast country.

While we were still thinking about our plans they both returned at different times so that was the end of that trip but we had other plans and that was figuring out when I could retire as I was feeling the on set of chronic 'burn out' and I had no desire whatever to keep working into old age and my dotage.

Partnership

When GP Ken Junior returned from Australia he decided to work with me for a year and that certainly was great news particularly when he suggested that he would continue the rota with Don so that I would have no weekend work and only one night per week on call. He also suggested that we would both carry on sharing the surgeries. I was really thrilled with this arrangement so Eileen and myself doubled our efforts to complete our retirement plans, which we did by the end of September 1989. We had decided to work one year from 1st October 1989 to 1st October 1990, which would be by sheer coincidence exactly thirty-five years since the day I started in Moville and to really round it off the 1st October would be a Monday so I would be off from Friday 28th September 1990.

I then started a countdown in every diary and calendar in the house and I could not believe that for that year I would only have to work for a few hours every day but in a very short time I felt that that was enough so I had no doubt whatever that we had made the right decision and at the right time to retire.

In the meantime Thomas had returned and himself and Cathy got married in May 1989.

Kenya

Early 1987

Eileen frequently mentioned that she would love to go on safari in Africa but we usually went somewhere else. Eventually one night I was reading either Time Magazine or The Readers Digest where I saw an article on famous train journeys like the Orient Express or The Blue Train in South Africa etc. It also mentioned the overnight train from Mombassa to Nairobi.

The words had a sort of a lilt as they tripped off my tongue. I then said to Eileen 'how does that sound?' and she replied 'great' and then I said, 'There is a safari thrown in as well' so that settled it.

My problem was mosquitoes as I had seen a man die from malaria.

We got ourselves well covered with injections and tablets a few months before we left. We then went off by KLM to Nairobi where we stayed in the Stanley Hotel for two nights and then went off through Nairobi National Park to begin the safari, which was to last for several days and finish up in Mombassa.

The roads had no real surface except a red dust and these roads stretched for miles in a straight line for as far as the eye could see. The transport was special types of jeeps and well protected from attacks from animals. The jeeps travelled in convoy in threes or fours and kept in touch with each other all the time as well as having frequent stops. They frequently stopped to check in case of accidents or other problems. They also stopped where animals could be viewed but we all stayed in the jeeps but could look out through the open roofs. At the end of the first day we checked into a hotel, which was really a complex of chalets, which were built like native huts and they included the old fashion type of muslin cover, which enclosed the beds. This area was known as the Kilimanjaro Safari Hotel.

We got out early in the morning to get a view of Kilimanjaro, which becomes covered in cloud later in the day. We were fortunate to get a view of the famous snow capped peak to take several photographs before the cloud descended.

Over the next few days we saw all the different animals wandering around the open spaces. The most common was the zebra with their black stripes. They travelled in herds and they appeared like donkeys. There were numerous giraffes eating the tops of trees along the roads.

We had a brilliant sight one evening of a line of several mother elephants with their baby elephants walking beside them on their way to a waterhole to drink. The safari ended in Mombassa where we stayed for a few days rest and swimming in the Indian Ocean. Mombassa was a very large town and was at one time was the capital of Kenya but in recent times the capital is Nairobi. We then left Mombassa to board the train for the overnight journey to Nairobi.

This was the climax of our visit to Kenya so we had no intention for sleeping for the night.

The train appeared to be very comfortable so we had a prolonged meal and then savoured the thrill of travelling through part of this vast continent. As dawn slowly appeared we could see more and more animals running away from the train in all directions as the dawn was turning to daylight.

We had a long day to wait in Nairobi for our return flight and then a few days of jetlag but with a large store of memories of our short experiences in Africa.

The Land of the Pharaohs

Aunt Alice and husband were in Cairo Egypt for several years but we have no recollection of hearing them mention anything outside Cairo.

It was a TV programme some time in the late eighties about Tutankhamen that stirred our imaginations. I remember a bit of history about Napoleon waging war in an Egyptian campaign confiscating some treasures.

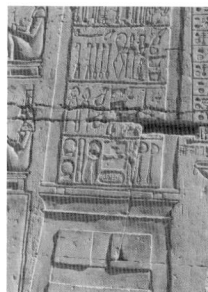

The pharaohs were obsessed with death and the after-world so they buried vast quantities of precious metals like gold, jewels, etc with the nobles and kings, which were nearly always plundered by robbers over many years.

When the English and French became interested they discovered massive temples and numerous treasures completely buried in sand and this opened up a new world of excavations, which is still going on.

In 1988 we decided to go on holiday to Luxor as this package had included a short cruise on the Nile we decided on Luxor rather than The Pyramids.

The large temples to various Gods were large buildings with massive pillars up to sixty feet high and thirty-one feet in circumference.

There was a spectacular theatrical show in a temple near Luxor called Karnak where these colossal pillars or colonnades formed huge temples.

This show in Karnak is known as the 'Son et Lumiere' (light and darkness) show. We were at this show on our first night there where all the spectators sat in a type of stadium in darkness. It was a calm balmy night with a full moon in a cloudless sky. There was a narrator describing each part of the temple as it became illuminated and dimmed in turn as the spectators walked around the huge columns. This was a moving introduction to our stay in Luxor.

In the temple of Luxor there are reliefs on the walls showing a birth room, also surgical instruments, and also depicting women giving birth in the squatting position.

We also visited the Valley of the Kings and Queens. Due to the extreme heat we travelled across the Nile at 6 am to avoid the extreme heat of up to 90 degrees.

Due to his early death Tutankhamen (1361 – 1352 BC) was not a famous pharaoh but he became very famous when his tomb was discovered in 1922 and the archaeologists found that it was full of treasures as the earlier robbers did not penetrate fully into the burial chambers. In that time in 1922 he became the most famous name in Egyptology. His body is now in some museum so people can walk down steps to the tomb.

Needless to say Eileen and myself went down. Paintings on the walls of the tomb were as fresh as when they were put on three thousand three hundred years ago. I have the treasured photograph of herself coming out the gate and another in deep discussion with the guide. This was the highlight of our tour except for a cruise on the Nile back to Luxor and later on a native boat called 'Felluca'.

We saw so many sights that could not be recorded here but we enjoyed our short time in Egypt.

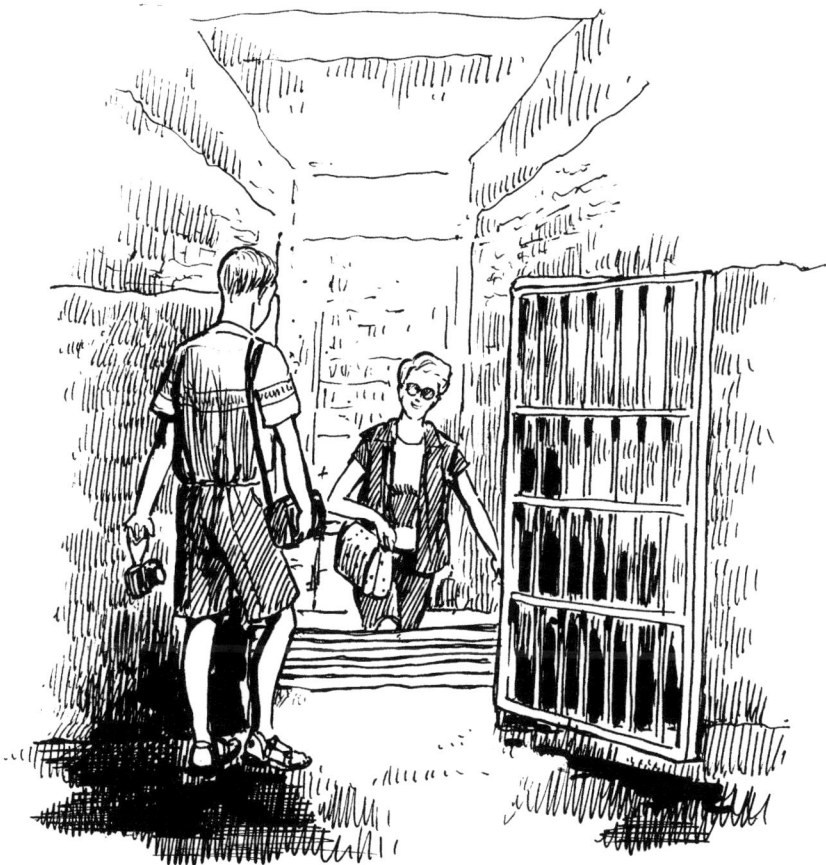

I.C.G.P.

Since the foundation in 1984 I was a regular attender at faculty meetings and never missed the faculty annual general meeting, usually held in March, when new officers like chairpersons, secretaries would be elected for the coming year.

At the meeting in 1990 there was some difficulty in obtaining a chairperson as there were no takers including myself, as I had never any desire to take on extra duties like this so I kept the head down. Eventually the chairman stood up and loudly stated he was leaving the chair and that Ken O'Flaherty would be the next chairperson.

I was seated on an end chair with my head still down until I was pushed out onto the floor. Like once before in the Coombe hospital the 'penny dropped' and I suddenly realised that I now had extra help in the practice and was about to retire in seven months so why not accept and enjoy the honour which unknowingly then was to lead on to the presidency of the college six years later.

Having accepted the chair I was requested to act as a faculty representative on the national council of the college. I declined the honour but reassured the meeting that I would accept it the following year.

As I was now chairperson of the faculty I felt obliged to attend the AGM of the college which is held every May. It is a large weekend gathering of members of the college with spouses and families in a large hotel with conference facilities also workshops, lectures etc. It is also a big social event and I certainly enjoyed my first meeting, which was held in Wexford. As I would be retired from all responsibilities of general practice I was looking forward to attending future meetings in changing venues all over the country.

Retirement

After the Wexford AGM 1990 there was now just four months to go to retirement so Eileen and myself were becoming very excited about how we were going to enjoy the new relaxed life.

According to our GMS contract three months notice was required by the health board but as I had no intention of or desire to do 'my own' locum as was customary in bygone days I decided to give four months notice. In writing it I stated that I was fully retiring from general practice on 1st October 1990 and that I did not wish under any circumstances to do my own locum either for a long or short term.

I had a very courteous reply from the health board thanking me for my letter and stating that they would honour my request regarding locums.

They thanked me for my work over many years and gave very best wishes for a long and happy retirement.

During the next few months I had separate visits from two health board officers to express their good wishes and to discuss my opinions on future manpower etc to be provided. My short reply was that at least three doctors were required.

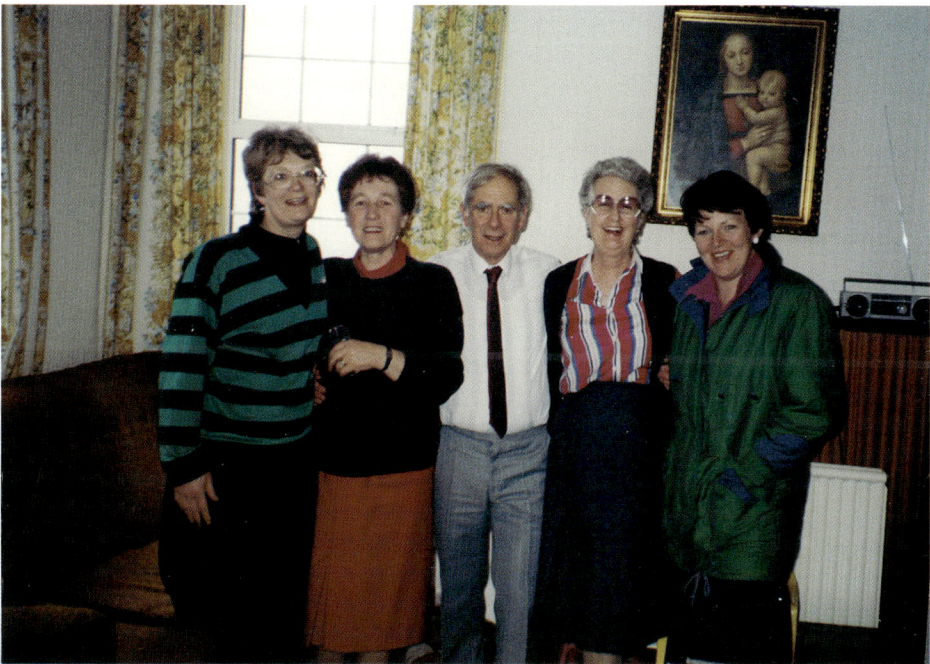

Phyllis Hasson, Greta, Ken, Nan McCarron, Mary McLaughlin, Ken's Retirement Day. (28/09/1990)

I put up notices in the waiting room stating that I would be retiring fully on 1st October and this included both GMS and private practice.

Most patients accepted and agreed that I had worked hard enough for a long number of years and that it was time I had a rest and a new lifestyle. I could never imagine myself seeing three or four patients per day which would necessitate changing from my gardening duds into a suit several times per day and continuing the stress of trying to get patients into hospital etc.

The summer of '90 moved on. Our second GP, Gerard, had graduated from Trinity and was starting GP training in Altnagelvin Hospital in Derry. Ken Junior was all set for going to New Zealand for a year. Thomas was working away in Windmill Lane; so all three were self-sufficient. We had missed Australia but we were now free to go to New Zealand.

The Light Keepers

As Inishowen Head was a land station and for many years three families lived in the dwellings provided on the station so there was a movement of light keepers and their families all the time. There were also several keepers living in the Greencastle area who worked in stations around the coast.

It was a happy coincidence for me that my earliest memories of Ballyconneely were keepers coming and going to Slyne Head. Later I had attended keepers as patients in Monkstown hospital in Dun Loaghaire and eventually having the honour of being their official medical officer for thirty-five years. I remember delivering at least one and probably two babies in the Inishowen Head dwellings.

Of all the keepers I had met one man stands out in my memory and that was Danny O'Sullivan a native of Whitegate, Co Cork a place that is also familiar to me from the time I first met my wife to be in 1954.

Danny had come to Inishowen Head many years before I arrived to the area. He married a local lady and made their permanent home there.

When we first met I am certain that the first question I would have asked him would be 'Have you ever served in Slyne Head?' My first impressions were that he was a highly intelligent person and a real gentleman.

He was a brilliant naturalist, a poet and author and he must have set a record by writing an article about nature for The Irish Press entitled Land and Water six days a week for forty-five years without a break. He won the Poetry Ireland award in 1980 and the 'Wilham Allingham' prize in 1983.

He had three sons who were light keepers, Hugh, Eugene and Donal and also at least one brother, Eugene senior, who served in Slyne Head. He married a Clifden lady and settled there. He was friendly with my brother Bernard and in later years they played golf together on the Connemara links. Ironically they both died suddenly around the same time in 1994. Eugene junior had the sad honour of being the last man to leave the last manned Irish lighthouse 'The Bailey' in Howth Head when the whole service had become automated in 1990.

A short time before retiring I notified the Irish Lights Head office of my intention to retire. On receiving my letter the following morning the chief officer phoned and informed me that the Irish lights ship the Grannuaille was on its annual inspection tour with the commissioners on board and to mark my retirement invited me to join the ship a few days later at Moville when she would be on her way up the Foyle to visit Derry.

From Slyne Head to Malin Head, A Rural GP Remembers.

I was thrilled with this invitation, which would be a fitting end to my 'Odyssey' from childhood in Ballyconneely through Monkstown Hospital, the tour on board the Irish lights ship the Isolda in Dun Loaghaire harbour and thirty-five years Irish Lights Medical officer in Moville.

On a calm September morning the Grannuaille arrived off Moville where a launch was waiting to take on pilot Dan McCann and myself to board her. As she sailed up the historic Foyle I recalled the hot afternoon standing on the ditch near Ture when I vowed never to leave this place. I also mused on the history of Grannuaille herself and her stronghold in Bunowen Castle when she was married to Dhonal 'Na Coga' O'Flaherty. My paternal grandmother was an O'Malley but no relation. (There are genuine descendants but certainly none in our family).

After a sumptuous buffet lunch in pleasant company the ship returned down the Foyle and left me ashore at Moville.

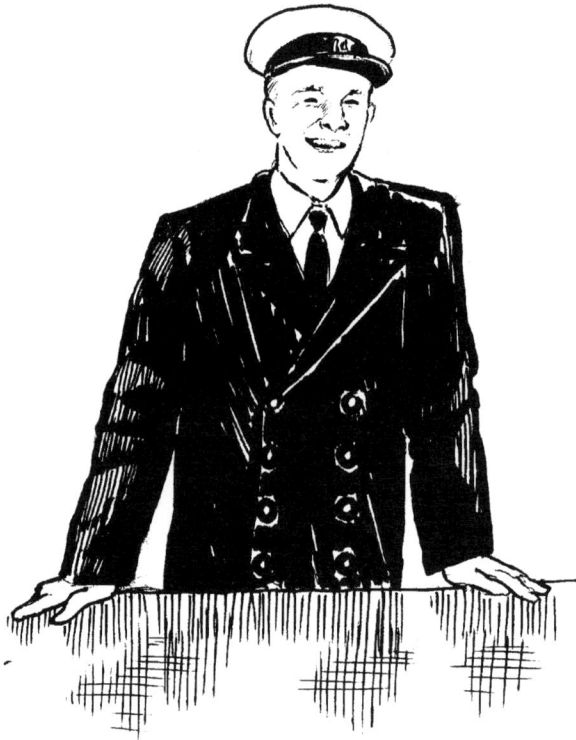

From Slyne Head to Malin Head, A Rural GP Remembers.

28th September 1990

As the retiring day drew near there was an air of excitement. I had planned to stop work at 4 pm on that Friday and I had arranged that as few patients as possible should come as I had arranged for the filing cabinets and files to be taken away that afternoon to a temporary surgery in the dispensary where Nan was now to change over to Don's practice.

We had already taken photographs of our staff including Greta, past practice nurse, Nan, present practice nurse, Phyllis Hasson and Mary McLaughlin the two district nurses (community nurses).

There was a sort of an open house and the few patients that came in were invited inside for drinks or tea and more photographs while Ken did whatever calls were required. It was a relaxed but also an exciting day.

As the time moved on to the 4 pm deadline and when Nan put up the sign that Don was on duty a patient came in who required to be nebulized.

The patient left at 4:15 pm and that was the end of thirty-five years of general practice, which with all its ups and downs gave me great satisfaction and above all I was grateful to the good Lord who allowed me to survive to enjoy a happy retirement. My feelings that evening were of great celebrations and relaxation like the first day of school summer holidays, passing the leaving cert, graduation, wedding day, arrival of new born babies and all other celebrations rolled into one.

Eileen, myself and the two sons who were nearer home went out for a meal that night. Ken was all set to travel to New Zealand on the following week.

Follow up Celebrations

On Monday 1st October Eileen and myself began preliminary enquiries with a travel agent about our proposed journey to New Zealand. For a long time we were walking on air and the preparations for New Zealand kept the 'high' going.

It was customary in Inishowen for the local GPs to organise a celebration party for a retiring colleague and this was held in late October. Our sons presented us with a voucher for a six-day holiday between Ashford and Dromoland Castles. The final celebration was the big public night in the Parish Hall.

The Pool

During my last year working I had changed from running to fast walking plus cycling in the summer months. I was playing tennis for a while but had to give it up due to a back injury.

The important thing was that I was keeping up the fitness and much to our delight a large indoor heated pool was built in Redcastle Hotel.

This was no Mickey-mouse pool. It consisted of a well-heated large adult pool plus a very good sized children's pool plus a small gym plus a sauna, steam room and Jacuzzi.

This pool opened just a month before we retired and we could not believe our luck in having this facility just six miles away in which we could 'wallow' every day and better still they had reduced membership for seniors.

Our routine from then on was to go to the pool roughly on five days weekly and swim non-stop of thirty minutes followed by a spell in the sauna and steam room and finish off in the Jacuzzi. This was really brilliant on the dark miserable days of winter.

We really enjoyed the remainder of 1990 looking forward to the trip to New Zealand. While I had made a complete cut-off from all medical practice I was still chairperson of the I.C.G.P. faculty and with no worries or stress of working I enjoyed the monthly meetings in Letterkenny and on the journey home I gloated on the fact that I had no worries or problems about the next day's work!

New Zealand

At the end of January 1991 and the start of the Gulf War we set off for New Zealand. On these long haul journeys to the other side of the globe there is a choice of one long direct flight to your destination or breaking up the journey with several stopovers usually two or three day breaks in order to see other parts of the world.

We arranged with our travel agent to have stopovers in five locations, Singapore, Hong Kong, Tiwan, Tokyo and on the return journey around the other side of the world, Fiji. The sheer size of the documentation in the itinerary was awesome and I wondered where it would go wrong but all credit to our travel agent Deirdre McBride everything went according to plan 'almost'.

At the end of January we set off in the BMW on a Monday morning to drive to Belfast International Airport on route to London Heathrow. As we reached the top of Glenshane Pass the car stalled a few times and then cut out. Our only hope was that the car could run down the long hill towards Maghera and could possibly restart and much to our relief this is what occurred.

Fortunately we had several hours to spare, as our flight from London was not until that night so if the worst happened we could have phoned the private garage at the airport where we always left the car. When we did get to the garage we informed them about the mechanical problem and requested them to sort it out while we were away.

We departed from Heathrow that night on a thirteen-hour flight to Singapore. This flight was longer than normal due to a diversion to avoid the Gulf War zone.

As everybody agrees Singapore is a very pleasant and clean place with a warm climate. We enjoyed the Chinese cooking in the famous outdoor restaurant in the famous Newton Centre. This was a great experience having left behind a miserable January.

Hong Kong and Mr Wong

Our next stop was the old world famous romantic city or territory of Hong Kong. We landed at the old airport where the aircraft had to fly up a street between skyscrapers when landing and taking off.

Our short stay there was a fantastic experience. Having seen many pictures over the years it appeared familiar when we got there. The sheer mass of people crowding the streets especially in the evenings was astounding.

My sister Carmel had a stopover there when going on holiday to China and she had bought some clothing material from a man called Stephen Wong. She gave me his address card to find him if I wished to buy a tailor made suit which would be made in a few hours. After landing in Hong Kong I reckoned that I would never find this man's shop with the mind boggling masses of small shops, streets salesmen and thousands of signs in Chinese hanging from the buildings.

On looking at his card by some freak of observation on the miniature map I noticed that his address was very close to the hotel just a few minutes walk away so off we went on foot to Mr Wong's but despite much persuasion I did not buy a suit as our luggage was already overloaded and it was early days in our holiday but I did order a made to measure silk shirt which I collected an hour later. It is a wonderful memento of Stephen Wong.

Another experience was a tour in a boat around the area where many of the old inhabitants lived all their lives in junks, boats and barges. We were told that some of them never left homes even for a brief visit to dry land. They were known as 'the boat people' and it is possible that this culture had now changed. Our visit to Hong Kong was a very memorable experience.

Taiwan and Turbulence

The take off from the single run way in Hong Kong was not quiet the 'hairy' experience of the landing.

It was much faster as it just skimmed over a bridge and headed for Taiwan for a short stopover of one night and part of a day in the capital, Taipei.

We landed there in thick fog and pouring rain. After a long trip from the airport it was still raining the following morning and as we were due to fly out in the afternoon our options for sightseeing were extremely limited. Fortunately I remembered having a great interest in the communist revolution in China. When the Chinese leader general Chiang Ki Check retreated from the communist armies and took refugee in the offshore island of Formosa and changed the name to Taiwan much to the annoyance of the Chinese government up to the present day. Having this interest we opted for a short morning tour to see the huge heritage centre built to the memory of Chiang Ki Check by money contributed by Chinese supporters from all over the world. With our limited knowledge we enjoyed the tour.

Flight to Tokyo

In the afternoon we travelled the long distance to the airport. It was still raining and the fog was becoming more dense so we began to wonder if the flight could take off and did not relish the thought of staying another night in Taipei in the incessant rain and to make matters worse I had a sort of foreboding!

The flight did take off into the fog but it appeared to me to be climbing very slowly with a lot of vibrations. I was watching some of the cabin staff who were seated nearby and they appeared to me to have remained seated for a longer than usual time. At this stage there was some turbulence and then mayhem as the aircraft lurched over to one side causing the overhead lockers to open and the contents to fall out. The aircraft then lurched to the other side with the same result. I had my eyes closed and was quiet convinced that the plane was breaking up and that this was the end.

It then went nose down for what seemed an age probably a few seconds it again lurched to each side and then to a normal position.

During the upheaval I was convinced that we were going to crash so I rushed a few prayers and then began to think that as we did not appear to be very high we would hit the sea in a very short time and in my mind I could see the headlines in the daily papers the following day 'Plane missing over east China Sea'.

When we recovered we could see the state of the cabin with locker contents, papers and magazines all over the floor.

A man seated two seats behind us found his spectacles on the floor of the seats in front of us. This man reassured us that he frequently experienced this type of turbulence in parts of the U.S. The captain also reassured us.

The remainder of the flight was normal but we were very much relieved when we landed in Nariti airport in Tokyo. It was a cool frosty night, as we would have had at home at the end of January.

Tokyo

When we arrived at the hotel we found the staff extremely efficient and courteous and spoke perfect English. The bedrooms were extremely small but fully equipped. We found our room was like a caravan this is to save space.

One of the bars in the hotel was called the Fifteens Bar or room and the décor was made up of Irish and English rugby teams who played club or international matches against Japan.

On the first morning we were directed to join a tour of the city and before boarding the coach the group were photographed.

We were very impressed with all the overhead trains and highways. The parks and temples were very impressive. In addition to tourists there were large numbers of local people worshiping, praying and lighting candles at various Buddhist alters. We also visited a ceremonial Japanese tea party where everybody sits around on the floor. We did not enjoy the Japanese food particularly the raw fish dishes so we frequently went for fries in McDonald's.

On our tour we also visited the Tokyo Tower, which was built on a style of the Eiffel Tower but not as spectacular. On being transported to the top of the tower by lift we had the experience of the Japanese culture of packing people into trains and lifts. When the huge lift appeared to be packed tight many more passengers were manually pushed in tightly. The weight was no problem for the lift, which got to the top at high speed.

There was a good view of the large area of the city and the spectacular view of mountain Fuji the highest mountain in Japan.

New Zealand

Up to this stage all our flights were on Singapore airlines but on leaving Tokyo we boarded a New Zealand airlines flight bound for a ten-hour flight to Auckland on the other side of the world. On boarding the aircraft two things struck me the first was that the cabin crew were mostly men and they were certainly mighty men, their heads almost scraping the ceiling of the cabin and their width filling the aisle. They could have been all retired from the 'All Blacks'.

The other thing was a very pleasant surprise, we were ushered into the first class seats where there is much more room for stretching legs.

We queried this but were reassured that they were our seats. We were already excited about this being the last leg of our journey to New Zealand and we now had the bonus of this luxury.

It was an overnight flight so we landed in Auckland on a brilliant summer morning. It was really a wonderful experience to have landed on the other side of the world on such a beautiful day. We still had to connect with the flight to Napier where Ken was to meet us and take us to his flat in Hastings where he was working.

There was a slight hitch in the itinerary which entailed waiting until late afternoon to connect with a small plane holding about fourteen passengers and made several stops at very small local airports on the way.

We had assumed that we were to connect with a normal jet, which was a half hour flight we were still very happy to wheel our luggage around in the sunshine outside the terminal.

One of the small airports on our way was in Gisburne the locality where the sun first shines on the earth on each new day. When we eventually landed Ken was there to greet us and take us to Hastings. He had taken a holiday so that he could drive us around the North Island and we had arranged a coach tour of the South Island when we returned. After a few days rest we set off on our tour of the North Island. On the first day we visited the Lake Taupo and the nearby Mount Tongarriro where it was possible to drive up to a summer resort, which became a ski resort in the winter.

We stayed overnight at Lake Taupo and did a tour on this large lake the following morning. There was a very big volcanic eruption in Mount Tongarriro in recent times. We then went northeast to Tauranga and the east coast where there were beautiful beaches with warm springs under the sand, which came up over our feet when we wriggled them in the sand. We then moved north to tour around the Coromandel

Peninsula where the scenery is magnificent and then back south to Rotorua famous for its sulphur springs producing the pungent smell of water on ashes.

We then went back to the east coast, then south to the East Cape and followed the coast to Gisburne and along Hawkes Bay to Hastings.

We enjoyed the North Island immensely. We stayed in small motels each night as these were scattered along the scenic routes. The climate was like the Mediterranean but probably not as hot in the summer. There were masses of forests and foliage of every description all different species of fruit were growing in abundance. The numerous large lakes produced electricity and the numerous hot springs provided hot water.

After a few days rest in Hastings admiring the beautiful Sam McGready rose gardens and other species of magnificent flowers Eileen and myself headed off on a service bus to join the Newman's Tour of the South Island in Wellington. There was one thing we could never contemplate and that was driving a car in a foreign country.

South Island

The coach tour officially started in Wellington where we met tour officials and other tourists. We stayed the night in a hotel for an early start the next morning to board the ferry to take us across the Cooks Straight and the scenic short cruise along Queen Charlotte Sound to Picton where we boarded the coach to take us around the South Island.

Our driver and manager was named Tony Ward and was no relation to Ireland's former great out half. The tour went down the west coast, which was slightly similar to Irelands west coast with plenty of drizzle. The mountains were much higher and many of them had glaciers. Over half way down the coast we went inland to Lake Wanaka and then to Queenstown, a large inland resort on Lake Wakatipu. This lake is unique in that there is some sort of preservation order on fishing so the lake is full of fish that can be seen in multitudes just under the water and are very partial to bread.

Bungee Jumping

It was near Queenstown that we saw the craze of the early nineties, bungee jumping. The coach driver asked the passengers, in general, if anybody had seen bungee jumping. Nobody had. He then turned off the main road and travelled a short distance to where the act was. The jumping was from a disused railway bridge at a great height over a gorge where the fast flowing white water was just visible at the bottom. The jumper was fastened to a rope, which was in turn fastened to a spring or some sort of elastic type rope called the bungee which slowed down the fall and brought it to a halt just over the rushing water a long way down near the bottom of the gorge so close to the water that a person in a rescue craft could just reach the dangling body and get him or her into the rescue boat and on to a landing stage.

Most spectators agreed this was a terrifying experience to watch. During that period it was a minor industry in Australia, where it was invented, and in New Zealand. When it reached Ireland it was much less terrifying as the jumping took place from cranes due to the lack of deep gorges in this part of the world. I imagine this pastime has died out by now but I am not certain.

We moved on from Queenstown along by Lake Wakatipu on to another scenic area in Milford, which is really a fiord but not anything as spectacular as the Norwegian fiords. We then pressed on to Invercargil where we passed through a frightening thunderstorm and flooding which fortunately did not last very long. This area is the most southerly part of The New Zealand mainland.

A few miles further south we visited Bluff the actual most southerly point in the territory of New Zealand which includes Stewart Island south of Bluff, either way the next stop would be the Antarctic.

Mount Cook

From Invercargil we travelled north east to the university town of Dunedin and then north to O Maru and then north west to visit Mount Cook the highest and most spectacular mountain in the southern hemisphere after Kilimanjaro in Tanzania.

We were very fortunate in reaching the small beautiful resort close to the mountain during a spell of warm dry weather. As with all very high mountains their peaks are obscured by cloud most of the time.

We arrived in the afternoon and were really thrilled by the spectacular views of this enormous mountain with its snow-capped peak and huge glacier which gave us the perception that we were almost beside it.

As we walked along the Hooker Valley, near the mountain, we were spellbound beholding this awesome sight of mountain, snow and glacier enhanced by the clear sky and evening sun.

At intervals we could hear loud rumblings and a cracking noise which was caused by large chunks of ice breaking off from the glacier.

We were all informed, that night, that the views of the rising sun on the snow-capped peaks should be very spectacular. In the morning when dawn arrived we were all waiting and certainly not disappointed when the rays of the sun hit the snow-capped peak. The magnificent reddish colour moved up the peak with the rising sun. When the spectacle ended I had used two rolls of film capturing this memorable experience, in what was to be the highlight of the whole tour. We have a treasured memento of a small painting of the mountain and the valley.

On leaving Mount Cook we returned by Lake Pkaki and on to Lake Tekapo to have a last view and take photographs of the distant peaks and then travelled north east through the Cantubri Plains to Christchurch where the coach part of the tour ended. Christchurch appeared to be very old and clean city and appeared to have been built to a definite plan as all the streets were in parallel lines. There was also a man-made river going through the city.

We stayed for one night and then got a train, early the next morning, which brought us on a very pleasant journey, northward. Along the coast to Picton where we got the ferry to Wellington and then the service bus to Hastings where we rested for two days before starting the long journey home.

The Long Journey Home

We began with a very short half-hour flight from Napier to Auckland on a jet, which connected, with a flight to Fiji, which was the last of our stopover flights, which would be going from west to east to complete our circuit of the world.

We had three very relaxing days soaking up the tropical heat, swimming in the lukewarm water, and the Polynesian hospitality and culture.

We departed from Fiji at 8 pm on a Saturday night and after crossing the Dateline and six hours flying we landed in Honolulu at 8 am on Saturday morning or was it still 8 pm or what?

I remember when studying geography that 'going west a day goes west'. We had to leave the plane and remain in a transit lounge for some time before taking off for Los Angeles and then another wait in a transit lounge before taking off for the ten-hour flight to London Gatwick. While on long haul flights I am always intrigued by continually following the flight paths as projected on the screens.

As we reached the south coast the path went up the west coast and then went east across Inishowen, which unfortunately was covered, by thick cloud. We then realised that we had completed the circle of the world despite the fact that we had yet to land in Gatwick, fly to Belfast and then drive the ninety miles to Ballybrack.

When we arrived in Belfast we collected the keys and we were all set for the last leg of the longest journey.

Let Down by the BMW

Life is supposed to be full of surprises and when the BMW refused to start we certainly got one, which at first sounded like a minor detail, requiring a touch of the jump leads. We had not forgotten the peculiar way she was acting before we left home and we thought she was only joking on top of Glenshane when she sprung to life on the way down the hill and why worry we had the car park garage to put her right!

When the jump leads did not work a few garage men took over and pushed, shoved and towed her up and down the forecourt making several forays under the bonnet without success.

It was eventually decided that the problem was probably a fault in a computer enclosed in a sealed box which required a specialist BMW mechanic who could not be obtained until the following day (Monday).

Fortunately the garage company had also a self-drive business so there was no problem making an arrangement for us to hire one and return it in a few days to one of their staff, who could collect it in Derry where he would have the BMW.

We were certainly relieved to take possession of the self-drive and get going on the motorway as soon as possible. After a short time the father and mother of jetlag set in like a general anaesthetic. You can just about imagine how much jetlag could be accumulated between Fiji and Belfast but we were determined to press on regardless by changing driving every fifteen to twenty minutes until eventually we got to Ballybrack Moville and the longest journey had ended. All that was required now was to stagger into bed.

The jetlag gradually wore off after a week and we were glad and relieved that I did not have to get back to real work in fact it was one thing I could not contemplate. This had been really a trip of a lifetime and as I write ten-years later it is still a very happy memory.

Between the great excitement of retiring and then organising the holiday with the travel agent 1990 had come and gone and we had reached March 91 and about to get back to real life. As we settled down, we now had all the time in the world to work in the garden with no more rushing, time to enjoy walking; swimming in the pool and Eileen had her golf, which she enjoyed so much.

Mental Health Association

In March 1991 I was invited to join the newly founded Moville and District Mental Health Association, which was founded in February 1991, and covering Northeast Inishowen. It is affiliated to the Mental Health Association of Ireland but is completely independent from it.

Its main aim is to promote good mental health as well as providing assistance and support to those suffering from or recovering from mental illness. Also to break down the barriers of a certain amount of stigma yet attached by society to those who have suffered or still recovering from mental illness.

The founders were a group of very enthusiastic and dedicated people spearheaded by Mrs Maura Cannon from Culdaff, Co Donegal. While the association is an independent body it liaises with the North Western Health Board whose community psychiatric nurse gives great assistance and advice.

The association has various ways of breaking down the barriers in the community. The most popular method for everybody is the social evenings, which are organised by association members, relatives or recovering patients and voluntary helpers. Music and singers are also provided.

The socials are held in various Parish halls on Sunday afternoons in the winter months where there is great intermingling and enjoyable time is had by all.

The association also hosts educational seminars on mental health issues. Other activities include visiting patients in the hospital or their homes, providing transport and assistance for attending Moville Day Centre.

Another very important activity is involvement in the mental health of Ireland public speaking project for secondary school students.

This is a type of competition where the students have to research subjects related to mental health issues and speak for three minutes on their chosen topic.

This appears to be an excellent method of very large numbers of students nationwide obtaining a basic knowledge of mental health which at least some of it would be shared with relatives and friends.

Origins of Serenity House

From the early days of the association it was agreed by the membership that a respite home was a necessity. Great efforts were made to purchase a suitable building but without success until 1997 the association, in partnership with the North Western Health Board, purchased a large seafront house: 2 Montgomery Terrace, Moville. Initially to be used in a respite facility for careers of those with mental health problems.

With a change in government policy carers are enabled through grant support to arrange their own respite.

Serenity House has expanded towards to becoming more broadly community based whilst maintaining its mental health purpose at present a wide variety of programmes and facilities are offered there by a dedicated and enthusiastic staff.

Serenity House is now a large resource centre for the whole community with a fully equipped computer suite, photographic dark room, audio visual library, conference rooms, computers, fax and typing service, various educational courses and active retirement programme for people over fifty-five.

I was an active member of the association from 1991 – 1995 and was chairperson for two years. I resigned in 1995 when I became vice-president of The Irish College of General Practitioners. I feel very honoured to have played a very small part in the association for a short time. I am thrilled for the association in achieving and expanding the original goals.

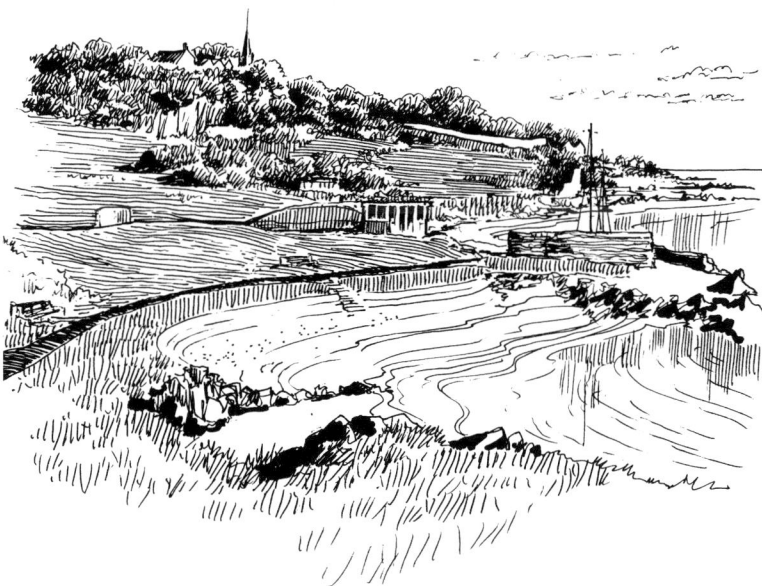

From Slyne Head to Malin Head, A Rural GP Remembers.

Promotion in the ICGP

In March 1991 I was re-elected chairman of the Donegal faculty of the ICGP and representative on the national council. This was an interesting and very pleasant appointment, which involves attending the annual general meeting of the college, which was held in the month of May in a different large hotel every year. Every faculty in the country had at least one representative and some large faculties had two. There was one meeting at the end of the AGM, another at the end of October and one in March.

Eileen always travelled with me and she enjoyed playing golf with other spouses on the Saturday of the weekend.

I was a faculty rep for seven years, which I enjoyed very much particularly on returning home on a Sunday night.

At the end of a council meeting I had no worries about starting back to work on Monday morning or worrying about problems that may have accumulated over the weekend. This was the beauty of having the best of both worlds when retired!

Bungy the Westie

Eileen and myself had a great love for dogs and during our early years in Moville we made three attempts to have one but something always went wrong between a fatal disease in one incident, postmen and patients complaining about being scared, by being attacked and barked at etc etc. We gave up the idea of owning a dog until we retired.

It is a well-known fact why dogs bark at postmen and not doctors. This is because the postman normally approaches the door, drops the mail through the letter box or just inside the door or under the door and then goes away quickly so the dog gets the impression that he or she is not welcome so his instinct is to hunt them away.

When the doctor arrives he or she is welcomed into the house and worse still is brought to a bedroom either upstairs or downstairs so the dog accepts him or her as part of the family.

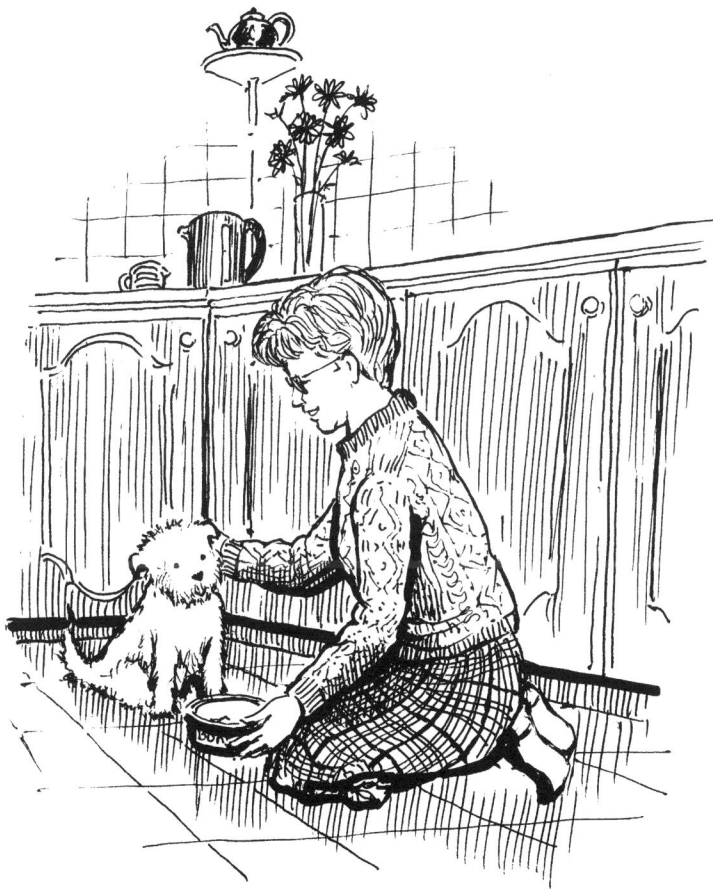

From Slyne Head to Malin Head, A Rural GP Remembers.

My routine in visiting a house for the first time was to make friends with the dog and just in case of any mistaken identity I always held the medical bag at a strategic position between the dog and myself. Over my thirty-five years in practice I was bitten twice.

One was a definite case of mistaken identity by the dog because while I was very familiar with the family where a long terminal illness had recently ended I had rushed in the open door to get directions to another house while the dog was sleeping in the sun outside the open door I was not carrying the bag and he got his teeth into a superficial bite on the back of my leg.

A second bite was from a vicious dog that was lying under a table growling at one side of the kitchen while I was 'rooting' for something in my bag with my back to the dog. When he stopped growling I relaxed while he crossed the floor quietly and gave me a good bite on the back of my leg. His owner, a bachelor living alone, had him out the door very fast and locked in an outhouse. Needless to say whenever I visited that house again the dog was well locked away.

Before leaving for New Zealand we had decided to get a dog on our return and had arranged with a local dog breeder to keep us a male West Highland from a litter that would be due in March 1991 and by May we had a two-month-old 'Westie' who is now eleven years old. Our first pleasant duty was to choose a name so I began to think of places and incidents that we had experienced in New Zealand and the first thing to enter my head was bungy or (bungee) jumping so he was duly christened Bungy or Bungee.

The Rise and Fall
of Donegal GAA

When we came to Donegal football in most of the county particularly in Inishowen was soccer while Gaelic was mostly played in the southern region of the county. This situation was due to the fact that Glasgow, due to emigration, was a hinterland of Donegal and vice a versa it followed that many parts of Donegal particularly Inishowen support for Glasgow Celtic was fanatical so that not alone was GAA excluded but there was no interest in southern Ireland soccer either.

The infamous GAA ban also played a large part in this situation and when the ban was eventually lifted both soccer and Gaelic benefited.

Meanwhile in the early seventies Finn Harps, a junior soccer club, based in Ballybofey was admitted to the southern Ireland senior status and in 1974 won the FAI senior cup. While the club has not been successful in recent years they have retained their senior status.

Our three sons and myself were at that famous cup victory when a Donegal team had won a National title. We had been regular fans since their foundation and we have great memories of that final.

Meanwhile the Donegal Gaelic team were improving and in the early eighties won an under twenty one All Ireland title. In 1983 they won an Ulster senior title to reach an all Ireland semi-final, which they lost to Galway.

We were at that match with mixed feelings but would have been happy if Donegal won. That was the day we saw Eamon Coughlan win the world five thousand metres title on the big screen in Crooke Park. The picture was coming from Helsinki.

The Donegal seniors came back again at the end of the eighties and early nineties. I was fortunate having weekends off from between 1987 – 90 and as I was retired in 1991 – 93 there was no problem in attending several Ulster finals between Donegal, Tryone and Derry. At this time our son Gerard was working as a junior doctor in Altnagelvin Hospital and most weekends off so he did all the driving. These were very close games until eventually Donegal defeated Derry in the 1992 Ulster final in Clones and went on to defeat Mayo in the semi-final.

We were at that match in Croke Park and despite the match being a very poor one it was really brilliant for Donegal supporters, who were all thrilled by the fact that the county had reached an All-Ireland Final for the first time. This was to be against

Dublin who had won well over twenty All-Irelands, a few less than Kerry.

From that day until the final the excitement in Donegal mounted day by day and as the day approached colours and bunting appeared everywhere.

By coincidence on the Friday before the final I was representing the Donegal faculty of the ICGP at the opening ceremony of a new orthopaedic department in the general hospital in Letterkenny.

It was a fine September day, which brought out the green and orange colours on every pole and gate.

There were flags in every house as well as slogans wishing the team good luck. Lorries, buses, and every other form of transport were all bedecked with the colours. The main street was crowded with people selling hats, scarves and flags; one could have been looking at Clonliffe Road or Fitzgibbon Street in Dublin as the town was awash with colours, excitement and good humour so that the sheer mass of expectation and willing the team to win was very palpable.

When the opening ceremony in the hospital was finished and the guests moved on to the dinning room for the buffet and speeches the atmosphere was brilliant with another mass of colour decorating the tables and walls. I have an abiding memory of that day in Letterkenny. Unfortunately I could not get a ticket for the match but I made the most of the T.V cover except for the awful blunder that a commercial took over when the Donegal team ran on to Crooke Park to contest their very first All Ireland final.

The result is now history but the victory celebrations had yet to come as the historic journey with the Sam Maguire Cup was made by train from Dublin across the Shannon and to Sligo, then by road to Bundoran where the Sam Maguire was carried ceremoniously across the Drowes River (which separates Donegal from Leitrim) by Brain McEniffe trainer or manager of the team and the captain Anthony Molloy to enter the county at Bundoran and then the triumphal journey across the Erin at Ballyshannon, eventually to reach home in Donegal Town well into Monday morning. That Donegal team reached two league finals in the following two years and lost two more Ulster finals by very close margins. If their luck had lasted they had the potential to win another All-Ireland but that was not to be.

The Rock Hill 10K (6.2 Miles)

As the triathlons and fun runs became more competitive after 1986 I kept on cycling in the summer months and also swimming and fast walking. In 1992 a charity run, combined with a walk, was organised by the army personnel stationed in Rock Hill in Letterkenny and was known as the Rock Hill 10K.

In 1993 I was still involved with the Moville Mental Health Association. In association with the organisers of the 10K in that year the Moville Mental Health Association were nominated as one of the main beneficiaries of the 10K charity run and walk. A large number of members of the association worked very hard to canvas many volunteers to take part in the 10K as runners or walkers.

I was delighted to be involved with this and thrilled to be able to take part in the walking section where I felt I could finish in a good position even in the first ten or twenty. The walk and run were held in the month of May so I trained very hard at walking over the next two months.

This was normal fast walking not the crazy walk inflicted on real walking athletes.
The Rock Hill 10K started at the army base south of Letterkenny. The course for the several hundred participants went towards the town then along Pearse Road to the roundabout at the bus station then along the Derry Road and then a left turn onto the Ballyraine Road past the Errigal Hotel then left up the hill and down the other side and then on to the main street and back to the finish at Rockhill.

At this time I was feeling very fit and I was looking forward to taking part in this walk with so many enthusiastic people especially all my colleagues in the Mental Health Association.

The Run and Walk

The runners went off first and then the walkers I felt very comfortable with my pace despite some difficultly with the crowded start. As the walk settled I could see four athlete walkers, two men and two women, well in front and moving further ahead until eventually they moved out of sight. As the walk went on I could see that the only people ahead of me were walkers who were running on and off and would not be considered in the competitive part of the walk.

As we approached the finish I began to think that I could be in fifth place but I seriously doubted that it could be possible. About two hundred yards from the finish I got a sudden tearing sensation and pain in the lower part of the calf on my left leg, which brought me to a sudden halt and the horror of having torn or ruptured the Achilles tendon. Despite this apparent disaster I could see that there were no walkers going past me so I just sort of dragged the injured leg side ways to the finishing line. With the assistance of some Red Cross personnel I could verify for myself that the tendon was not ruptured and better still I was informed by an official that I had finished fifth over all but as there was a male and female category I had finished in third place in the men's category and that the official time was one hour and twelve and a half minutes for myself this was an overwhelming achievement at sixty-six and a half years of age.

While I was counting my blessings, a long standing friend and former professional colleague of mine, Seamus Temple, a psychiatric nurse, came to my aid and assisted me into my car and instructed me to follow him to his nearby home where he could apply an ice pack to the injured muscle.

I was most grateful for this great attention and I certainly enjoyed the cups of tea while watching part of the Eurovision Song Contest.

I managed to drive home with the ice pack in place in time for the end of the Eurovision, which as far as I can remember was won by the Irish representative, Naoibh Kavanagh.

I was back again for the 1994 Rock Hill 10K well aware that while I would enjoy the competitive walk again I was not going to be in the first five but I actually finished around ninth or tenth. That was to be my last walking, running or cycling event, as we will see later.

ICGP Council and Wonca

During those years from 1991 I was enjoying retirement more and more and being a member of the college council was a fantastic experience to be part of this body of dedicated people striving to develop and improve the standards of general practice. At this stage it was just seven years established so it was an exciting time to be part of its organisation.

This enthusiasm was demonstrated when in 1992 the college made a successful bid to have a world conference of general practitioners in Dublin. This world organisation has the title of WONCA, which is defined, as the 'World Organisation of National Colleges Academies and Academic Associations of General Practitioners'.

WONCA is held every three years so in 1991–92 the Irish Council, decided by a very large majority vote, to send a delegation to the WONCA conference in Vancouver that year to make a bid for the 1998 conference to be held in Dublin.

They were successful in their bid so from 1992 until 1998 WONCA was on the agenda of every council meeting and every AGM. I found it a fantastic experience to be on the council for all those years.

There was also another very important recurring item on the council agenda and that was the obtaining of new premises for the college headquarters as the existing rented building was becoming completely inadequate for the increasing workload of running the college.

These two big projects were just a small part of the overall workload of the college staff which included the main work of the college in communicating with all the faculties in organising research projects, ongoing tuition in various subjects to mention but a few items and above all the annual preparation of the college membership exam, training ancillary staff like practice nurses, secretaries, practice managers etc etc, also assisting faculties in organising AGMs. All this workload and more were required to assist GPs in keeping up to date. During all this time the secretarial and administrative staffs were working under extreme pressure due to lack of space.

Death in the Family

At the end of February 1994 Eileen and myself went on holiday for two weeks to Tenerife. We were enjoying the sunshine and heat every day and the nightlife in the hotel every night.

At the end of the first week we were looking forward to the second week. That evening as we were at dinner I was paged to go to the reception. As I walked the long distance from the dinning room to the reception I was full of foreboding and as I reached it I was directed to a phone and when our son Thomas introduced himself I said immediately 'who is it?' and he replied that Bernard had died suddenly on his local golf course that morning. Thomas had phoned the hotel several times during the day but we could not be located as we had been out all day. As Bernard had a by-pass operation in 1987 the shock was slightly cushioned but at 8 pm on a Saturday evening getting home on time was the real worry. Despite having insurance for such an emergency wondering where to start was the big problem. We started looking up the tour operator's book near the reception in a sort of panic. Fortunately a tour representative, who was off duty, observed us and enquired if we were in trouble and if she could help which she certainly did.

She suggested that she would start phoning from our room so we all went there and within a very short time she had contacted the travel insurance and put us on to them. They explained there could be difficulty on a Saturday night and Sunday morning but they would phone back as soon as possible. After half an hour they had phoned and said that they had arranged a flight on Iberian airlines from Tenerife at 6 am to Madrid to connect with a flight to Heathrow, to connect with a flight to Dublin and that we could collect our tickets at the airport.

We then phoned Thomas and gave him the time to expect us in Dublin. Everything went according to plan. We had first class tickets and while waiting for the connection in Madrid airport we were shown to the VIP lounge.

Tom and his wife Cathy met us at Dublin airport and brought us to Bernard's home in Kilmessan, Co Meath, where we arrived before the removal.

Our travel insurance was one connected with our credit card and we were very impressed with the courtesy and efficiency of their handling of the journey.

They did not demand a death certificate or any evidence to back up our claim. Our travel agent put in a claim for recouping part of our holiday expenses and we received payment without any problem.

The Doctor Patient Again

After the 1994 Rock Hill 10K, I continued walking, cycling and swimming in the pool also mowing the grass and gardening as usual. At the end of September I noticed a pain in my left knee joint, which gradually became more severe so I had to give up the cycling.

At the end of October I had difficulty in walking and had to use a stick and worse still I had severe pain at night. In desperation I made an appointment with one of the orthopaedic surgeons in Letterkenny General Hospital.

He told me that I had no cartilage in one side of the joint so surgery was necessary as soon as possible. On a dark wintry morning at 8 am on 1st December 1994 I was wheeled into the theatre and some time later wheeled out with my left leg from foot to groin encased in a plaster cast. Fortunately this was the modern scotch plastic type of plaster, which was very light compared to the old plaster of Paris.

This cast was to remain on for seven weeks so I was supplied with crutches. The great thing about this was being retired and having no hassle obtaining locums.

The other bit of good fortune was the time of year, which was similar to the time I was off with TB in 1950. December and January but this time I could do three miles daily on the crutches up and down the path where I most have clocked up hundreds of miles running and fast walking over the years since 1983

Re –Hooked on Joyce

When I first got hooked on Joyce back in the sixties I eventually got to read his portrait of the artist and Dubliners. At some stage one of my sons gave me a present of Richard Ellmann's biography of Joyce a tome of some 744 pages. Now was the time to read this great work which was hard going but worth the trouble.

Joyce's world famous book Ulysses is not a book for reading on a train or plane journey. It required real study to get some understanding so I started by studying Tim Severin's book on the voyages of Ulysses and then a book by Harry Blimer on how to read and get a basic understanding of Ulysses. I read it four times so I reckon that I could have a 'juvenile' knowledge of Joyce.

Stunned

On Sunday morning in early January 1995 I got a phone call from Michael Coughlan who was then the chairperson of the ICGP council. Without beating about the bush he told me that at an executive meeting of the council on the previous day it was decided to offer me the vice-presidency of the Irish College. I was really stunned by this and nearly fell off my crutches! So I replied, 'Hold on until I discuss it with Eileen' and he replied by telling me to phone back in ten minutes. Eileen and myself decided that we could not refuse such an honour so I then phoned Michael that I had accepted.

The protocol is that the proposed vice-president is installed at the next AGM, which by a coincidence was to be in Bundoran in May 1995, and on serving a year as vice-president I would be installed as president the following year, which would be in the Tower Hotel in Waterford in May 1996.

The ICGP Presidency

The ICGP presidency is very much an honorary appointment and the main duty is to represent the college at social functions of other related medical or paramedical organisations. He or she also attends various forms of medical conferences like book launches etc or other in-college functions like conferring ICGP membership diplomas and various academic prizes at AGMs. The president did not get involved in medical negotiations with the Department of Health. The chairperson usually carried this out. The vice-president becomes a member of the executive of the council for three years, the first year as vice-president, the second as president and the third year as ex -officio. The vice-president carried out the same duties as the president when required to assist so that he or she could be very busy at certain times and as a member of the executive was expected to attend six executive meetings in the college headquarters in Dublin in addition to the normal three council meetings held at different venues throughout the year. While I was still in the plaster cast and on crutches I was trying to come to terms with the honour I had received and could not figure out how it happened. I was really thrilled and in addition there was the excitement of being involved in the organising of the coming AGM in Bundoran.

This involved extra meetings and sixty mile journeys on icy roads to meetings in Donegal Town where we would meet with college staff who would have travelled from Dublin.

We also had extra local meetings in Ballybofey. While I was in the plaster cast Eileen did all the driving as well as having to drag me out and pull me back into the car! She had driven to a council meeting in Dublin and back during the snow until our luck ran out and we had to change a wheel in the dark near Omagh. I had many years' experience in changing wheels but not with my leg in a plaster cast. Just as I began to grapple with the task a young man in a car noticed our predicament and came to our rescue. To get back to earth after the New Year excitement I was looking forward to having the plaster removed and just dying to get back into the pool.

When it was removed everything was satisfactory but I now had the task of getting the knee joint to work again, as it was stiff as a board.

So after two days I got back to the pool, which was a fantastic experience to be mobile again in the water without the aid of crutches.

After half an hour continuous swimming using the good leg and putting pressure on the stiff knee I knew I had the perfect 'physio'. On emerging from the pool I would go to the steam room to put more pressure on the joint by pulling for 10 – 15 minutes on the leg and measuring the distance that I could pull back the foot on the floor tiles and note the improvement every day. I had a similar session in a hot bath at home every night so that after three weeks I had almost got full flexion.

I gave up the cycling but resumed walking at a normal pace using a walking stick. I have continued the swimming even though some biased rheumatologists and orthopaedic surgeons would blame athletic activities for causing osteoarthritis. If they are correct so be it! I never had any regrets about my years of running and cycling. With a family history of generations of heart attacks I would prefer to have osteoarthritis and I never had the slightest regrets that I resumed running after my illness in 1975 when I was forty-nine years of age and walked 10K (6.2 miles) at sixty-six and a half years in seventy-two minutes

Life in the ICGP Fast Lane

While still in the plaster cast, and later recovering from the surgery, I was attending faculty meetings and AGM organising meetings and all this activity was boosted by my being the vice-president elect of the college. Eileen and myself were thoroughly enjoying ourselves, as time was our own. The months from January to mid May moved rapidly to our big weekend. Despite cold weather and hail showers there was also some sunshine in that memorable weekend in Bundoran.

As incoming vice-president I was experiencing a certain amount of V.I.P. treatment with photographs and interviews, which ended at the council meeting on Sunday when I was given the chair and inducted on to the executive so as one roller coaster ended I was starting on another as we headed back the eighty miles to Moville taking the scenic route by Rossnowlagh to have a meal in the 'Smugglers Creek' restaurant.

During my time on the executive the college was all the time improving tuition facilities for members, bringing in newer courses etc. for newer skills it was also coping with three huge commitments.

The first was the mammoth organisation for WONCA, which was now only three years down the line.

The second was the purchase of the building of an adequate headquarters.

The third was the planning of a national survey of general practitioners.

As vice-president the first duty was to attend the executive meetings and to assist the president in office carrying out his or her functions. When duplicated and when really pressed the ex-officio president could step in.

The main function was to represent the college at annual dinners of other medical or paramedical organisations. At these functions the vast majority of people were out to enjoy themselves and so were we. Spouses attended most functions so Eileen and myself never missed anything we always enjoyed being led to the top table where there was always laughter and banter. The presidency was really spread over three years as the vice-president had to perform very frequently for the first two years and very occasionally in the third year.

Our first big function as vice-president was to attend the conferring ceremony of the membership diplomas to the new college members. This was held in the Royal Hospital, Kilmainham, which is a very impressive heritage building.

Our next duty was a very exciting and historic day. We were invited by the Royal College of Physicians in Ireland faculty of public health who were hosting their first ever-scientific meeting in Northern Ireland in the City Hospital to attend the meeting and to be guests at a banquet to be hosted by the Lord Mayor of Belfast in the City Hall on that night.

This was on 30th November 1995 the day that Bill Clinton visited Belfast for the first time while still president of the USA.

As a result of the president's visit the Lord Mayor had to change his plan and host the president of the USA and his party in the City Hall. So the medical dinner was changed to the Stormont Hotel.

This also changed our plans, as we could not travel on our normal route to Belfast due to the massive security so we had to take the long way around to reach Belfast from the eastern side.

We stayed in the Wellington Park Hotel, which was near the City Hospital so there was no problem in attending the meeting. The banquet went ahead with a massive presence of US security men all over the place in the Stormont Hotel and kept up the excitement of the day that was in it.

We were invited to the residential weekend of the Royal College of General Practitioners Northern Ireland faculty: October 1995, in the Killyhevlin Hotel, Enniskillen, in October 1996 in the Slieve Donard Hotel Co Down, and in 1997 the Radisson Roe Hotel in Limavady the nearest place to home as we can see the lights of Limavady across the Foyle at night.

We were also invited to a conjoint meeting of the RCGP and ICGP in the Killyhevlin Hotel, Enniskillen in April 1996. This meeting had invited the president of the Royal College, Mrs Lottie Newman and her husband Norman. She promised at the time that she would attend our AGM in Killarney in 1997.

At the end of January 1996 we were back to Belfast. Bill Clinton was gone but snow had arrived so we decided to go on the bus from Derry, as we were to have a very busy weekend.

This time we were invited to the annual dinner of the Ulster Medical Society, which was held in the Great Hall of Queens University. We checked in at the Wellington Park again as it was in a short walking distance from Queens. It was snowing at this stage but it cleared when we started to walk.

The dinner was the start of our weekend agenda as we had planned to attend a council meeting in Wicklow on the following day so the plan was to travel early by train to Dublin and the Dart to Wicklow and the Glen O'Downs Hotel for the council meeting. One of our sons was in Dublin and would take us home if the snow cleared in time. As usual we enjoyed the banquet in Queens and walked back to the hotel wondering how the snow would be in the morning. It was no worse so we got an early train to Dublin and eventually got to the Glen O'Downs and the council meeting and back to Moville on the following night.

In 1997 we were back again in Belfast for our second dinner in Queens but by this time I was the full president.

We were invited to numerous functions north, south, east and west while vice-president and to many more when president, while many would be repeat invitations the following year.

We enjoyed every minute of the vice-presidency as we were free from real work. The working president delegated a considerable amount of work to us, which really whetted our appetites for more so we were looking forward to the presidency, which approached very fast.

When the time arrived we decided to take two days for the journey, as it was a long trip from Moville to Waterford. We stayed in Gort for the first night and as the weather was good we made the short trip, the next morning, to visit Coole Park, which was once Lady Gregory's home where she entertained Yeats, Oliver Gogarty and other literary luminaries. We then went on a leisurely journey to Waterford to the Tower Hotel and the AGM.

AGM

The AGM consisted of a weekend from Friday afternoon to Sunday afternoon. There were several workshops and lectures on topical subjects of the day. Spouses and children were encouraged to attend while organisers and hotels catered for children's activities.

There is usually a buffet super and cabaret on Friday night and the annual banquet on Saturday night. On Sunday morning the AGM takes place and chaired by the outgoing president when it ends the outgoing president hands the chain of office over to the new president who then gives a short address 'to the multitudes' outlining his or her hopes for the continued success of the college. During my time in office the three main objectives were 1) purchasing or building a new headquarters, 2) the organisation of the WONCA conference, 3) the up coming GP survey. After the new president's address there was a photo call followed by a long address on a special topic by an invited guest.

The President from Donegal

While I felt very honoured by being invited to accept the presidency I had no doubt it was mainly an honour for the Donegal faculty, which was very enthusiastic from the foundation of the college and played a large part carrying out research projects.

In conjunction with the North Western Health Board, members played a large part in spearheading Cardio Pulmonary Resuscitation (CPR) training, which was a pilot scheme to be followed over the country.

The faculty really became of age when, despite a number of difficulties, it hosted the 1995 AGM in Bundoran.

Having finished the protocol of the changeover and instalment of the new president the next function would be the meeting of the new council. I was now the thirteenth president of the college.

As Waterford was only a short distance from Eileen's home place in Cork we had decided to stay with her brother, sister and family for a few days before heading for home.

We had a few days at home before setting off to attend several functions. The first was to represent the college at a lecture and dinner to honour a founder member of the Irish College who died a very short time later. This was held in the Royal College of Physicians in Kildare Street on the 21st May. This establishment was founded in the 19th century and many of the famous Irish doctors of that time studied there. The college is now used for examinations and conferring of degrees and also provides medical libraries etc.

It also accommodates the Royal Academy of Medicine which was founded in 1882 by the amalgamation of four medical societies each one having its own special educational meetings in the college. There are now twenty-two sections or societies. Membership is obtained by invitation to apply for membership to the council to be elected to membership or fellowship of the academy.

This meeting was my first function as president and after the dinner I was invited by the then president of the academy who was seated close by to apply for election to membership of the academy.

Having spent many long hours of days and nights studying for exams I had no problem whatever in accepting this fellowship without the drudgery of studying for any type of examination. Having carried out the formalities I was duly honoured with a very impressive certificate and annual diary and I purchased an impressive tie with logo. The next function was on the following night 22nd May and this was to attend the annual dinner and to the conferring of the Faculty of Public Health of the Royal College of Physicians.

We represented the Irish College at many functions in the historic building in Kildare Street over our year in office and we certainly enjoyed every one of them.

Our next trip was further away in the Silver Springs Hotel in Cork. This was the annual dinner of the Pharmaceutical Medical Representative Association held on the 25th May.

ICGP Confering July 19th 1996

There was one practical function every year that was carried out by the president of the day and that was the conferring of the membership scrolls on the candidates who had succeeded in the college exam. For some years this ceremony was carried out in the Royal Hospital in Kilmainham.

This was an old building, which was at one time, probably in the time of the Napoleonic Wars, a hospital for treatment of old soldiers. It had been refurbished in recent years and was now a well-maintained heritage building with surrounding gardens. It is situated in the area near Stephen's Hospital and Heuston Railway Station.

In 1996 it was a unique occasion for Eileen and myself as one of our sons was among those who were conferred with their membership of the ICGP in the Baroque Chapel of the Royal Hospital.

To add to the occasion it was one of those rare hot, sunny July days, which certainly enhanced the old surroundings and made it a day to remember.

Professor Per Fugelli and Joyce

From the early days of the foundation of the Irish College an annual scientific meeting was held in the College Of Surgeons. This consisted of several workshops, lectures and posters. For some years Astra Pharmaceutical Company supported part of the meeting and included a visiting professor to deliver a topical lecture, which was held in a large lecture theatre in the College Of Surgeons. This lecture was always chaired by the president of the day.

The thirteenth annual scientific meeting was on 23rd November 1996, which was my year in the chair. The lecture was to be delivered by Professor Per Fugelli a professor of social medicine in the university of Oslo. Before starting the lecture I had asked him if he had been in Dublin previously and if he knew much about the city. He informed me that he had read about Joyce and mentioned Joyce's section in Ulysses about bloom and the 'shenanigans' of the students in the residency in Holles St. I wondered if many of the people in the lecture theatre knew anything about that episode in Ulysses.

After the scientific meeting we went on visiting venues hosting functions these included Castle Troy in Limerick and Great Southern in Galway, Slieve Russell in Cavan, Sligo Park Hotel, The Royal College of Surgeons in Dublin, McKee Army Barracks in Phoenix Park, several functions in the Royal College of Physicians in Kildare Street.

National Survey

In the year 1996/97 the big survey of GPs was on and I had been appointed as a type of enumerator in the Donegal faculty. This was to contact GPs who had not returned their forms and to remind them to get their form completed as soon as possible. This system was used in all the faculties and was very successful in obtaining valuable information for the college and the Irish Medical Organisation.

Our hectic year moved very fast and the next AGM was moving closer. Our last function was in the Hotel Westport which is in a town well known to me since childhood.

This was the Pharmaceutical Managers' Association Dinner. I knew a great number of the people there and we had a really great night of fun and laughter and what a befitting end to two years of an almighty roller coaster but there was still more to come.

Second AGM Killarney 9th – 11th May 1997

The AGM was a big time for the out going president between opening meetings, presenting and introducing political ministers and other VIPs and finally his or her speech at the banquet on the Saturday night.

My first council meeting in 1991 was at an AGM in Killarney Great Southern Hotel. That year it was all a new and exciting experience and it certainly never crossed my mind that I would ever return to this venue but after seven years on the council I was back again as an outgoing president and to really make this a very memorable occasion our life long friends Adian and Maura Meade were due to become vice-president on the Sunday afternoon.

Mrs Lottie Newman was still president of the RCGP. Herself and husband Norman had been invited when they had attended a conjoint meeting the previous year. Herself and Norman were delighted to accept the invitation to our AGM and also to see the beauty of Killarney renowned in song and story around the world.

Despite some inclement weather they enjoyed the traditional trip on the jaunting car and the tour of the lakes through the Gap of Dunloe.

Lottie was invited to speak at the banquet and brought 'the house down' when her opening remarks were spoken in almost fluent Irish. She had been tutored by Michael Coughlan, the chairman, some time during the day. This sent me into a spin to try and cobble together the 'cupla focials' to keep up with Lottie when I followed her speech so the bit of humour added to a very memorable night.

On the Sunday morning after chairing the AGM I handed over the chain to my successor Declan Murphy a former chairman and would be in office for the momentous year ahead which would include the hosting of WONCA in 1998 which was due to end on the 18th June 1998. There was to be no traditional AGM weekend but the basic protocol would be carried out on Sunday the 14th June. I would be in office as ex-officio until the 18th June, the day WONCA would end.

WONCA 98

Being a world conference of general practitioners held every three years it was a brave and mammoth undertaking to host.

When this great honour was won by negotiation high up in a mountain resort called 'Whistler' near Vancouver in 1992, preliminary work started under the guidance of the chief executive of the college Mr Fionán O'Cuinneagáin and gathered momentum over six years until June 1998. The actual date was set for the 14th – 18th June.

Back in 1992 the first problem was deciding on a venue, as there was no real international conference centre in Dublin. The nearest adequate centre was the RDS (Royal Dublin Society) in Ballsbridge. At that time the organisers where assured that there were plans for a modern international conference centre and it would be completed before 1998.

It is now 2002 and it has not yet got of the ground because of problems with planning permission. It was then decided by the organisers to use the RDS complex.

We were now in the last year of preparation for WONCA and still searching for a new headquarters. Suddenly an opportunity arouse when a developer offered a site in Lincoln Place which was just a few yards from the old offices in Fenian street and it was a prime site in the city centre. Work was to start in October 1997 and be completed in April to May 1998.

This deal was certainly a huge relief for Fionán O'Cuinneagáin and his staff whose working conditions were by now becoming intolerable.

As executive meetings were held in the old building in Fenian Street many GPs had a good knowledge of the conditions.

As I was at the last executive meeting in Corrigan House the old headquarters on 7th March 1998 and the first meeting in Lincoln Place on 9th May 1998 I had the unique distinction of experiencing the contrast between both venues in a space of two months. Early in 1998 the official information and program about WONCA arrived. The dates of the conference were confirmed to be from Sunday 14th of June to Thursday 18th of June in the Simmons Court Pavilion in the RDS. The program had arrangements for several tours in Dublin and environs and a vast number of coaches were drafted in from around the country to provide a continuous shuttle service from all the booked hotels to the conference site. There were several receptions to be attended.

Very much to my delight there was a tour to the Joyce Tower in Sandycove and the organisers made the most of the fact that Blooms Day (16th June) fell on the Tuesday of the conference, so there was to be a massive Blooms Day dinner and dance in the main hall of the RDS that night. There was also a talk during the conference lunch break delivered by the expert himself, David Norris.

I was highly excited and thrilled at the opportunity of the tour to the Joyce Tower and to attend the Blooms Day dinner and ball.

At the lunch break on Blooms Day there was an Irish recital on the fiddle by the senior paediatrician in Letterkenny Hospital, Dr. Seamus Maguire. Having studied the social program I immediately booked the tour to the tower and the Blooms Day Ball.

We had already booked into Jury's Custom House for the duration of the conference almost a year previously because we were free agents and determined to miss nothing! With the shuttle service, transport would not be a problem.

The Five Days of WONCA

DAY ONE

Early on the Sunday morning on our forty-second anniversary, 14th June, (that date is also the anniversary of the date that Joyce and Nora Barnicle met in Nassua Street while June 16th is the date of their first date) we boarded the coach with a mixture of several nationalities but we were the only Irish 'tourists'.

When we reached the tower the weather was bright and breezy and as Joyce described it there was a 'snot green sea' visible across Dublin Bay to Howth.

I immediately joined forces with Japanese and American delegates taking numerous photographs. I had waited a long time for this opportunity and I was going to make the most of it. We then moved inside to see the real 'life' scenes where Joyce and Gogarty lived for such a short time and where their friendships broke up.

I was surprised that there were no notices forbidding photography inside the tower, so I photographed everything that came in sight.

On returning from Sandycove to the conference centre the sun was shining and several delegates were having lunch or picnics on the grounds, shuttle buses were arriving and departing continuously as the numbers of delegates were increasing steadily and the 'buzz' was becoming more palpable.

There was a gigantic marquee, which housed numerous coffee shops, snack bars, pubs and kitchens. In the main building there was a mammoth reception and registration desk.

There were several small kitchens and snack bars. Banners and flags of the visiting nations were hanging from the ceilings, numerous lecture rooms and workshops. There was a large auditorium where plenary sessions were held and also used for the opening and closing ceremonies.

Before the opening ceremony we attended the ICGP official reception welcoming the president Mary McAleese. The president of the college Dr Declan Murphy welcomed her. After the formalities the president then addressed a very large number of delegates in the auditorium before officially opening WONCA 1998 which would really begin at 8 am on Monday morning.

The opening ceremony was then followed by a miming show by Macnas which was a very spectacular theme putting across the dangers of smoking. We had joined with

Aidan and Maura Meade and one of our sons Gerard and wife Siobhan and finished the night dancing to the music of Paddy Cole.

DAY 2

I was determined to enjoy this GP world conference without having any stress. I travelled on a shuttle bus at 7:30 am each morning to attend whatever lecture was being delivered by an expert from some distant country. This was followed by breakfast from one of the many kiosks and then leisurely tours around the numerous stalls and workshops, attending the occasional lecture and browsing around the huge area of posters displaying research projects by GPs from many different countries and cultures around the world.

As the weather was holding up it was a great pleasure to walk around the campus and take numerous photographs of the huge activity that was going on all over the place. There were many delegates rushing out, small groups having discussions in the sunshine others just relaxing. During each day of the conference I returned to the city to join Eileen for lunch and then both of us returned to Ballsbridge to enjoy the afternoon.

On the run up to WONCA the organisers had requested faculties to sponsor some form of hospitality for small groups of visiting delegates. As would be expected 'Donegal were on the Ball' so one of our hard working and enthusiastic members a very charming lady, Ms Karena Hanley, with other enthusiastic ladies organised a dinner and musical evening in the National Gallery Restaurant on the Monday evening where a number of Danish delegates were entertained.

The area near the National Gallery is a very historic area of the city. Oscar Wylde was born in Westland Row but moved at a very young age to the corner of Merrion Square, which is now the American College. Finn's Hotel where Nora Barnicle worked is also very close, as is Nassua Street where she first met Joyce and where they met for the first date was at the corner of Merrion Square opposite Wylde's home. The National Library where Joyce and Gogarty first met is also near.

DAY 3 TUESDAY 16TH JUNE BLOOMS DAY

On Tuesday I continued my early morning bus trip, which was interesting meeting delegates from around the world. I enjoyed the early morning plenary lectures as I am by nature a morning bird so the trip in the bus on mid-summer mornings was a wonderful start to the day. I regretted having to miss David Norris's talk and Seamus Maguire's music due to our lunch arrangements but we were not going to miss out on the Blooms Day dinner, which was a gigantic, gathering for eating and dancing.

DAY 4 WEDNESDAY 17TH JUNE

We were now approaching the end and the drizzle had arrived but we had to be thankful for three sunny days. However we were looking forward to a big reception in the home of the American Ambassador, Mrs Jean Kennedy Smith. The incoming president of WONCA hosted this. We were invited because I was a past president and still on the executive until the next day.

On the same evening there was a reception for all delegates in Dublin Castle, which was hosted by the government.

The Closing of WONCA 98

DAY 5 THURSDAY 18TH JUNE CLOSING CEREMONY

This was the closing day of WONCA so it was a half-day dealing with protocol and closing ceremony.

The incoming president from the US took over the presidency for the next three years until the next WONCA in Durban, South Africa. Michael Boland became vice-president and would become president of WONCA three years later in May 2001 in Durban. All this has now come to pass.

Michael Boland from Skibbereen was one of the many enthusiastic and dedicated GPs who founded the Irish College in 1984. His ability and enthusiasm was well recognised in the UK, Europe and other parts of the world. He is a full time director of medical education in the Irish College. Despite the lack of a modern conference centre in Dublin WONCA 98 was a success and had a record attendance of over 4000 delegates. This success was due to the college members who devoted many hours of work from 1992 – 98. There is one man in the highest echelon of the college who can keep a 'mind- boggling' amount of irons in the fire and with an encyclopaedic memory had the answers to any question fired at him, this is chief executive Fionán O'Cuinneagáin.

When the curtain came down to end WONCA 98 it also ended the minute role that I may have played in the council and executive over seven years. I had witnessed a great and exciting time in the college during those years, which has given me a large store of memories.

The QE2 1998

In early January 1998 I saw an advertisement by a travel agency offering a deal to Irish customers for a very reduced fare for a cruise on the QE2 from Dublin to the Arctic and back to Southampton. This deal included free travel from Southampton back to Dublin on the return trip. The ship was to call to Dun Laoghaire to take on the Irish contingent wishing to cruise visiting Iceland, Spitzbergin then Tromso, Trondheim and Bergin in Norway. The highlight of the cruise would be to cruise up probably the most scenic Fiord in Norway, the Geiranger Fiord.

Ever since that trip on the Mauretania from Cobh to Le Havre in 1958 we had frequently discussed our ambition to cruise on the QE2 now one of the last of the great liners built in Glasgow and would soon be on her way to a dry dock or the breaker's yard. This was probably our last chance to get such a bargain so in January we booked to join this massive ship at Dun Laoghaire on the 20th July 1998.

While we were both sun worshipers we were always wishing to go back to Norway

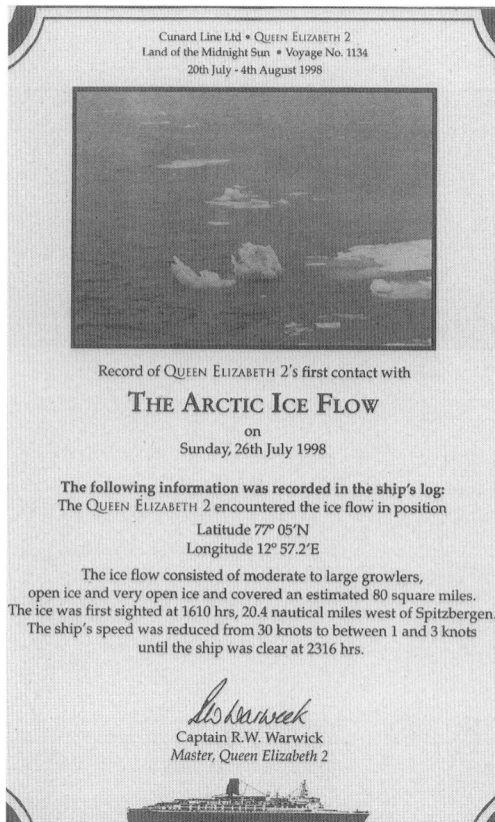

Cunard Line Ltd • QUEEN ELIZABETH 2
Land of the Midnight Sun • Voyage No. 1134
20th July - 4th August 1998

Record of QUEEN ELIZABETH 2's first contact with

THE ARCTIC ICE FLOW

on
Sunday, 26th July 1998

The following information was recorded in the ship's log:
The QUEEN ELIZABETH 2 encountered the ice flow in position
Latitude 77° 05'N
Longitude 12° 57.2'E

The ice flow consisted of moderate to large growlers,
open ice and very open ice and covered an estimated 80 square miles.
The ice was first sighted at 1610 hrs, 20.4 nautical miles west of Spitzbergen.
The ship's speed was reduced from 30 knots to between 1 and 3 knots
until the ship was clear at 2316 hrs.

Captain R.W. Warwick
Master, Queen Elizabeth 2

Holiday. (1998)

and see the midnight sun away above the Arctic Circle. When the day arrived it was typical July weather blustery winds and showers. We set off on a bus from Derry to Dublin then got on the Dart to Dun Laoghaire, then onto a launch to board the dream ship.

It was a fantastic thrill to get on board this old ship before her approaching demise, as we understood that a new ship was being built to replace her. That was four years ago so we have to wait and see!

After reaching our cabin the next chore is to get your bearings on the layout of the decks, stairs and lifts. On cruises food and entertainment is included and that means all meals, snacks, afternoon teas, buffets and helping yourself to ice cream from vending machines, all entertainment like stage shows and films are all included. As would be expected alcohol and cigarettes are not included and there is a large casino for gamblers. Use of inside and outside swimming pools are also provided.

That evening the QE2 sailed northwards along the east coast towards the North Sea and Iceland which we reached in a few days and went ashore in the capital Reykjavik. The weather was similar to our usual summer weather. We had a tour around the city and were shown how the natural hot springs and geysers are harnessed to provide central heating. We saw very large outdoor swimming pools where people can swim outdoors at all times of the year as steam can be seen rising from the water.

The old houses preserved as heritage show houses were similar to the original Irish homes/cottages, which had just 'scraw' roofs.

Spitzbergin and the Ice Flow

On leaving Reykjavik we went northeast crossing the Arctic Circle and on to Spitzbergin. The weather was now becoming colder similar to a cold March day in Ireland. We were due to arrive in Spitzbergin in early morning. There was no night as the sun did not set but it did not shine either.

I had set the alarm for 3.30 am to get up and experience the Arctic 'night'. It was full daylight but there was a haze or fog and the ship slowed down. When I reached the top deck, to get a good view, I noticed what I thought to be a boat, probably a pilot boat, coming out of the fog but as it approached the ship I noticed that it was a large lump of ice of several square yards in size, with the submerged part being a bright blue and green colour. Many more similar chunks followed this; I learned later the technical name was 'growlers'.

At this stage I was frantic with excitement taking photographs, climbing up ladders and reaching over rails to get better views. The ship was now crawling at about 2 knots to avoid damage to the hull. The normal cruising speed is 30 knots. During all this time more and more people were arriving on the decks to experience this Arctic annual phenomenon. We passed through this part of the ice flow in a short time as the blue and white masses of ice gradually disappeared astern.

We soon arrived off Spitzbergen and dropped anchor. It was cold here but not freezing. We went ashore in launches and 'moised' around the large wooden and well-heated shops where all sorts of fur and leather coats and hats were on sale.

Apart from the shops the island appeared rather desolate. The main or only other industry was coal mining, which was shared by Russia and Norway. I have no doubt that if the Arctic sun was shining it would have improved the scene immensely.

On returning to the ship we resumed our cruise to Tromso but after a short time we were back into the more dense ice flow so that the ship's speed was again reduced from 30 to between 1 and 3 knots, which was just a crawl so I was once more on deck photographing from all possible positions as larger 'growlers' appeared. These floating chunks of ice were quite thick so the submerged blue and green shades were now larger than in the early morning view. At this stage they could be heard and felt bouncing of the ship's hull.

By a strange coincidence the film shown in the cinema on the previous night was 'you have guessed it' Titanic this gave rise to a fact or a rumour around the ship that there were some elderly ladies, who were at the film, became somewhat disturbed about the ice flow.

Tromso

The reduced speed of the ship caused several hours delay to our next port of call, which was Tromso so that all the available shore tours except one had to b e cancelled. We were informed on the ship's bulletin that this was the first time the QE2 had encountered an ice flow.

When we arrived at Tromso at around 6 pm it was a balmy summer evening with many hours of sunshine yet to come. Tromso is situated at a very northern part of Norway so it must be very grim in the winter months. We went on the one short tour that was available to see a special type of film of the northern lights or the aurora borealis.

The remainder of the Norwegian part of the cruise was to be all sunshine and warm weather.

Our next port of call was Trondheim, which is a beautiful old Norwegian city and where we visited a ski jump site where the world ski championships were held a few years previously. While we were there we saw world-class skiers doing summer training on artificial slopes.

On leaving Trondheim the QE2 continued her journey overnight not to another port but to cruise up what has to be the most beautiful and spectacular Fiord in Norway, namely the Gieranger Fiord. On awakening we were just entering the mouth of the fiord on a beautiful warm sun-drenched day. The scenery of the towering mountains on each side of the waterway was magnificent. These mountains had a considerable amount of grass and foliage, which enhanced their brilliant appearance in the bright sunshine.

Up to recent times cattle were herded high up on these mountains in the summer months and occasionally some of the old houses or huts used by the herdsmen could still be seen.

As the ship progressed very slowly along this magnificent fiord most of the passengers were on the top decks spellbound at the magnificence of the changing scenery, occasionally small towns and villages appeared with winding roads ascending the mountains to disappear into valleys. Small aircrafts also called 'float' crafts fly in and out of the fiords landing and taking off from the water.

The waterway appeared to have gone several miles through the mountain ranges with frequent sharp bends for the ship to negotiate to reach yet another breathtaking view until eventually reaching its destination a beautiful resort around the shore at the end of the fiord.

We got ashore on the launch and had a wonderful evening wandering about taking photographs. A German man, who appeared to be alone, kindly offered to take a photograph of us sitting on a small wall with the fiord and ship in the background. It is now a very much-treasured memento.

As the evening approached we boarded the QE2, as her engines were revving up for our return journey back to the open sea, but as the night approached and the 'midnight' sun reached the horizon, brilliant new scenes arrived to paint the sea and mountains in a mixture of red, gold and bronze colours triggering off numerous cameras to click and buzz around the top decks.

The one photograph that I decided was my 'masterpiece' was a view from a passenger's small lookout deck near the bow and high up over the bridge of the ship. This photograph was of the sea as we left the fiord. In it a small boat was crossing the fiord leaving a narrow wake across a wide area between the mountains. What delighted me most was that I had not observed the small boat when taking the photo. By now we had left the Geiranger Fiord behind and headed south to Bergin, which we had visited in 1963.

The weather remained good while we were in Bergin but became cold and dull for the last leg of the cruise to Southampton to disembark and travel by coach to London to connect with the flight back to Dublin.

Thus our long held ambition of forty years was fulfilled.

Omagh

As I have attempted to record all personal experiences and other big events as far as possible in chronological order I feel compelled to mention the Omagh bomb, which occurred a very short time after the happy QE2 experience.

On that 15th August day I was reading the daily paper sitting in the car in a car park in Derry while Eileen was shopping. A newsflash came on the car radio that a bomb had gone off in Omagh but there were no other details.

Omagh is thirty miles from Derry and appeared to have been a quite relatively peaceful market town during the worst of the troubles so I was surprised to hear this news. A short time later another newsflash announced that there were some casualties and a large area was damaged. The next news bulletin had more details of the real horror, which killed twenty-nine people, and a busy shopping street almost demolished.

It later transpired that some young people from Spain, in Donegal on holidays, were involved; a young English boy living in Buncrana as well as two young Buncrana boys also lost their lives. In addition to the twenty-nine people killed there were very large numbers of casualties.

1998 – 99

After the excitement of WONCA followed by the QE2 cruise and then the horror of the Omagh bomb 1998 moved on to the official opening of the new ICGP headquarters in early December '98. As past chairpersons and past presidents are invited to all special occasions for life, Eileen and myself were there to celebrate this very happy occasion for the long-suffering college staff, and who did the official symbolic opening? You should have guessed, Aidan Meade who was president at that time. So forty-five years later after our first meeting in George's Street Dun Laoghaire in July 1953 we were all four still on track!

Health and Day Centres

During this year there was one event which concerned Eileen and myself and that was the official opening of a magnificent new building combining a health centre and day centre in Moville.

For a number of years previously GPs and health boards were rapidly leaving the days of the single-handed dispensary doctor and the old dispensaries behind and co-operating to build new state of the art health centres in many of the areas throughout the country. These health centres have modern facilities, and ancillary full time staff of nurses, secretaries and managers etc and at least two to three doctors.

Moville was no exception as Dr Jack Magnier's successor Dr Don McGinley and my successor Dr Geoff Bourke both played their part with the health board. They now had a three-doctor partnership with a part time assistant and a full professional ancillary staff.

When I entered medical school in 1946 it was the first half of the twentieth century and when I retired in 1990 at age of sixty-three it was the last decade of the century. I was delighted and very grateful to have survived to see the new century and millennium and to witness this great progress. As I am sure readers have gathered by now that I am a fanatical believer in handing over to the next generation when the time comes.

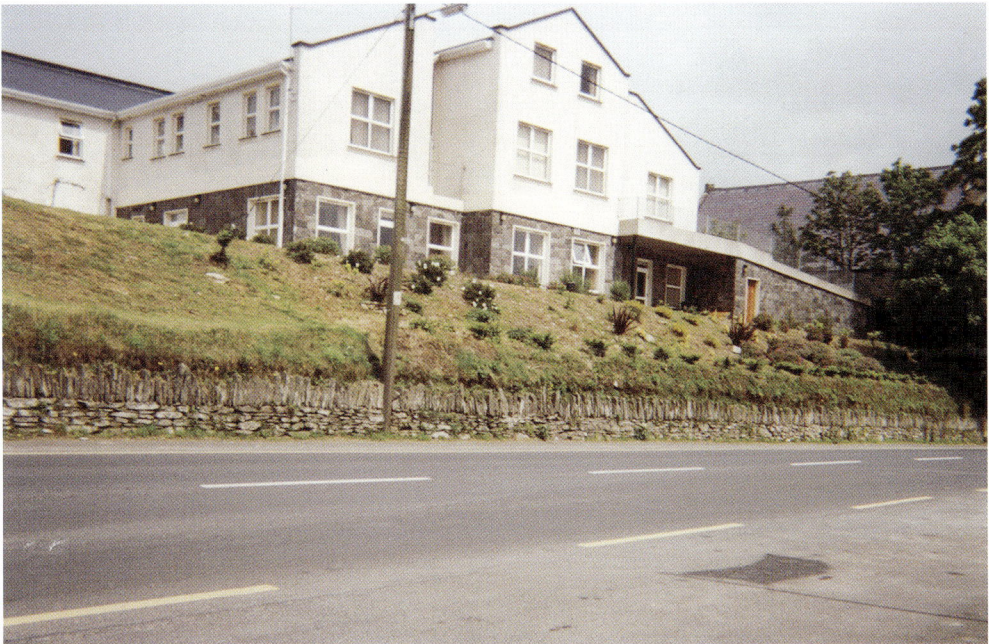

New Combined Health and Day Centre, Moville. (1999)

The combined health and day centres were officially opened in July 1999 by the then minister for health Mr Brian Cowan. Both centres were under the same roof and this co-operation of the day centre with the health centre was a fitting reward for all the work carried out over many years by voluntary workers since the foundation of the first centre in the old convent school.

It would be impossible to mention all those workers over the years but I feel compelled to mention three people who were prominent from the early days. One was my colleague, Dr Jack Magnier, one of the founders, who did a large share of work in the early years, another was my first practice nurse Greta Rawdon whose dedicated work and perseverance for the founding and early running of the centre, I personally witnessed for several years. Another was the long serving and dedicated Chairperson John (Vincy) Mc Laughlin.

Sadly Jack and Mary Magnier and Greta are no longer with us.

Eileen and myself felt very privileged to be still around and witness all these great changes.

The Millenium Bug

By September '99 we were rapidly approaching the end of the twentieth century. There was much media speculation about how to greet the new millennium but also concerns about computers 'going down' in various machines including aircraft, banks, cars, and even domestic fridges and freezers.

There were dire warnings and horrors of a sort of doomsday situations. All computer owners etc were instructed to have certain adjustments carried out. As far as could be ascertained probably most people carried out the instructions but certainly not everybody. It was also thought that aircraft would have to be grounded.

Workers in many occupations like restaurants and pubs were demanding vastly increased payments for working on New Year's Eve so then many owners closed for business that night.

The government supplied every household in the country with a special millennium candle to light on New Year's Eve at the moment of the last sunset, which was not visible in Inishowen due to thick cloud. It was visible at Dursey Island off the west Cork coast so we could at least see on TV and took photographs of the TV pictures. I had got excellent photographs of the sun rising over Benevena across the Foyle on the solstice (21st December).

The Millennium Spectacular

As midnight arrived in many world capitals each city produced real fiesta shows of massive displays of fireworks, native dress and dancing. They were brilliant displays and went on for several hours.

Sydney, Australia had an extra special show to celebrate the start of their Olympic year.

Granduncle Doctor
on Horse Back

I have in my possession a well-preserved leather bag containing several obstetric instruments, some orthopaedic and one instrument called a guillotine used for removing tonsils.

This instrument consisted of a loop of thin wire, which could be manoeuvred around the root of the tonsil and then the operator could control the loop to make a knot to pull out the tonsil. There was also a small brown bottle of chloroform and an anaesthetic mask.

All these instruments were covered with Vaseline and wrapped in newspaper and this has kept them in perfect condition. This bag was found in an attic in my mothers original home in the early fifties and it was probably used by her uncle who was probably a dispensary doctor around the Tuam area.

This was a narrow, rectangular, strong, leather bag with a strong carrying handle and appeared to have been a saddle bag which many rural doctors used when doing rounds on horse back in the early twenties or earlier.

Memorabilia

In October 1999 the Irish Medical Times had a notice in two or three of their weekly publications inviting readers to contribute articles or old photographs of medical buildings or other interesting objects for publication in a special millennium edition to commemorate the last century.

I took no notice of the first two requests but on the third notice I suddenly thought of my bag of instruments which were certainly part of the last century and possibly of the previous century. I got going very rapidly and rooted out the saddlebag of instruments and after some polishing of instruments and bag and numerous photographs; I mailed the photographs to the Irish Medical Times and to my great satisfaction my contribution was published in the special millennium edition in January 2000.

Mauritius

Eileen has a cousin Miriam who is a Loreto Nun. In the 1960's she was sent out to the missions in Mauritius situated in the Indian Ocean, east of the tip of South Africa. After many years there she returned to Ireland and later went to serve in the famine in Ethiopia for two years and then returned to Dublin for a while and was then sent back to Mauritius for three yearly stints with three months holidays after each stint.

During her holidays she always visited us, as she loved Inishowen. Every time she visited us she always asked us to take a holiday in Mauritius. We eventually made the decision to go and in September 1999 we booked a holiday to fly out on St Patrick's Day 2000.

When the day came we left Moville at 6:30 am to drive to Dublin airport. As it was St Patrick's Day the roads at that time of the morning had little or no traffic. As we left Moville we had the daunting thought we were now heading for the Indian Ocean and the tropical island of Mauritius on the other side of the world. Everything went according to plan and we were relieved when we reached Terminal 4, which is really an obstacle race. We had a smooth flight with Air Mauritius for the twelve hour long haul to our destination. It was wonderful landing into the tropical heat and getting into the warm sea.

We had a ground floor room about twenty yards from a beautiful horseshoe shaped beach with the green ocean protected by a reef so it was very safe for swimming. When we got a tropical shower, while on the beach, we just went into the sea and swam around until it was over. We would dry out after a few minutes on the beach. The dining room in the hotel had a roof but no front.

Miriam brought us to some lovely private beaches where we had picnics and great swimming.

The island is approximately twenty-six miles long and eighteen miles wide and she toured all over pointing out the sights. We also visited the schools and other places where the sisters did great work in helping deprived children from broken homes.

When she was there, in the sixties, the country was primitive but has developed rapidly in recent times.

While there was great poverty there before tourism was developed the new prosperity brought alcohol, drugs and AIDS so that there are always problems.

Sugarcane was and still is a big industry there but like other industries it does not employ the same numbers as previously. Originally the cane was harvested by labour but it is now mostly carried out by machinery.

Tourism is highly developed with new roads and motorways being built and there is a large extension and development of the airport.

There is a mixed population of African and Indian cultures. The island was occupied at different times first by the Dutch then the French and eventually the British. They all departed peacefully and the island got its independence when the British left.

While we were there, there was a cyclone alert when a strong cyclone originated in Western Australia at the start of our second week.

This cyclone was heading for Mauritius and as the danger approached everything around the beaches was tied down with ropes and all boats, of every description, were dragged out of the sea and lashed down. Tying down the loungers and chairs was no problem as everybody lay on their towels on the sand the same as at home. For the first three days of the alert there was no change in the weather apart from being cloudy and windy.

As Mauritius is small, cyclones usually miss it and this happened this time as it came close it diverted suddenly and headed for Madagascar. Miriam informed us that this diversion of the cyclones to Madagascar occurred so frequently that she felt sorry for 'poor' Madagascar as Mauritius usually escaped! While the alert lasted notices of direction and force of the cyclone were posted in the reception.

There was a high wind for the last two days and we were worried about possible delay of flights home but that did not occur. The only worry was an announcement by the flight captain just before take-off that as we would fly around the cyclone there would be some turbulence but not to worry about it. I was hoping that it would not be anything as bad as our experience over the East China Sea on our way to Tokyo in 1991. In actual fact we had no real turbulence on the whole flight and landed on time in Heathrow.

On leaving Dublin Airport we were thrilled at the bright spring morning and looked forward to a pleasant journey home. By the time we reached Monaghan the sun had disappeared and it was bitterly cold and when the Sperrins appeared they were covered in snow but fortunately the roads were clear. Once more we were very lucky because we met people later who could not get out of Belfast due to the snow.
We got home to a very cold house despite the central heating. Once more we were home and all that was required was to sleep off the jetlag in the happy knowledge that I did not have to get up for work the next day or any day. The only work was to get all the films developed and select the best of the photographs for the albums.

Carmel

Our generation of the O'Flahertys is a much smaller family than our parents' families. There were eight Lees and six O'Flahertys with just three O'Flahertys in our generation. Bernard the eldest, three years older than me and Carmel eight years younger.

Having no sisters she was very much on her own but she appeared to have a very close relationship with our mother. When Bernard and I went to boarding school she would have been starting the national school in Ballyconneely.

In the early days of the century, and up to the end of the thirties and later, there was a culture in business and large farmer's families that the eldest son would inherit the business or farm or both if they existed.

The next son or sons was destined for a profession or the church. The girls would be destined for the convent depending on their religion or they would be encouraged to do commercial training. On leaving the national school Carmel went to Loreto Abbey in Rathfarnham in Dublin. I was the least bright of the three of us finding maths and Latin nightmares but I still pressed on when I got the opportunity.

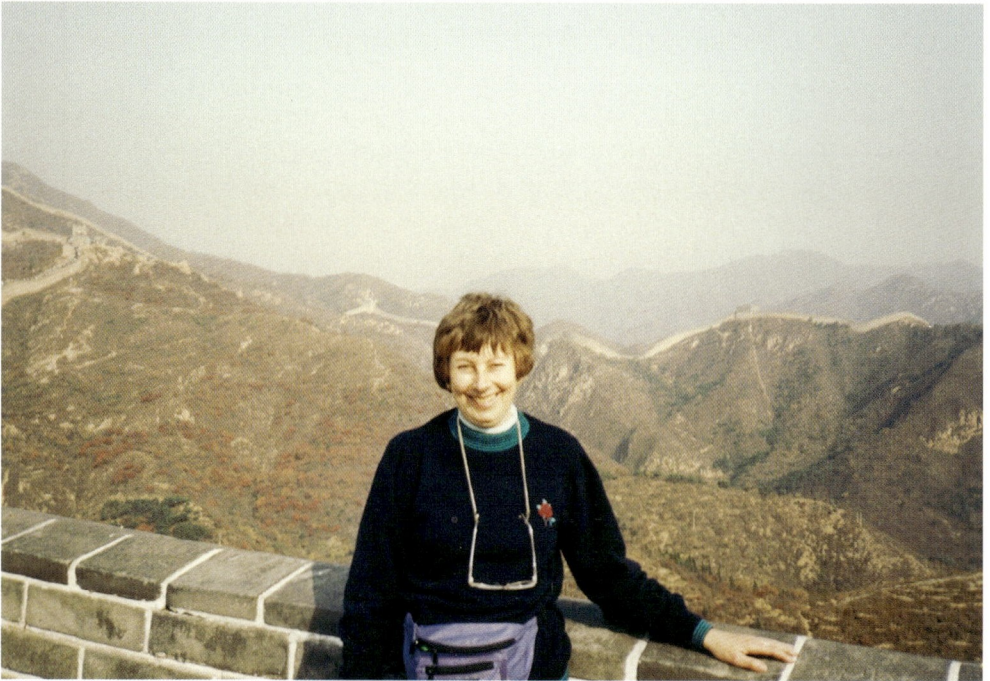

Carmel on the Great Wall of China.(1990)

Carmel was like the rest of us she loved sport and the outdoors. She enjoyed hockey and tennis when in boarding school and continued playing all during her career.

She would have been starting in Rathfarnham when I was in UCD. A classmate of mine also had a sister there so both of us used to cycle out to visit them on occasional Sundays. I have no doubt that Carmel more than paid back those visits when she visited our sons in Castleknock.

On leaving school she went to commercial college and on leaving there she spent four years helping out the business in Ballyconneely while our father was ill.

On returning to Dublin she worked in Jefferson Smurfit from 1962-67 at that time the company went public and became listed on the stock exchange. From 1967 until retirement in May 2000 Carmel worked in Bord Fáilte's head office in Dublin. She thoroughly enjoyed this job particularly in the last ten years when she was dealing with all sections of Irish tourism trade and also working closely with the board's overseas offices. This job took her each year on promotion work to North America and the UK.

While the schedules were gruelling she really enjoyed the events because of her love for travel. This work could involve covering a city with sometimes two promotions each day. This was physically and mentally tiring for all but the craic was also great.

Passion for Travel

Carmel's passion for travel took her to China on a personal trip some years ago taking in eight cities plus Hong Kong in three weeks. A few years later it was a trekking holiday in Nepal that covered nine days trekking/camping, three days white water rafting on the Triculi River, three days at the Chitawan Jungle Park, a two day stay in Phakhara and four or five days in Kathmandu, split between beginning and end of the trip.

During all these years she has played tennis and is a very keen gardener. In later years she does more hill walking at home and on the Continent.

Since retiring, Carmel has become actively involved in the newly formed Bord Fáilte Retired Association.

Throughout all this exciting and active career Carmel has kept in close contact with us all, chiefly with Bernard's family in Kilmessan, cousins in Galway and a cousin in America.

48th/50th 'Jubilee' Celebration
1952 – 2002

(To be celebrated on 48th anniversary to coincide with millennium year 2000)

As a result of a straw pole taken in 1998 it was decided to celebrate our class 50th Jubilee 1952 – 2000 on our 48th anniversary in the millennium year 2000 as it would give some of us a better chance of being still around in 2000.

That was the decision in 1998 so our faithful and stalwart organisers Aidan Meade, Una Comber Callaghan and Jerry Doyle got to work two years in advance of the date September the 8th – 10th 2000.

A programme was mapped out bookings arranged, addresses obtained and notices sent out. The final plan was a general social get together in the Berkley Court Hotel in Ballsbridge on Friday evening.

On Saturday morning a coach tour to Laytown Church to attend mass for deceased members followed by lunch in a local restaurant and then a tour to Newgrange. That night there was banquet in The Berkley Court. On Sunday there was an informal evening as guests of Aidan and Maura Meade with another group as guests of Frank Muldowny.

Millennium Reunion

Eileen and myself travelled to Dublin and stayed in Jury's Custom House and took taxis for transport to the hotel. We enjoyed the weekend immensely meeting so many classmates after so many years. We enjoyed the Mass in beautiful Laytown Church with its all glass gable facing the sea. Our late friend and neighbour in Greencastle, internationally acclaimed architect, Liam McCormick, designed this church and also designed our house in Greencastle.

We then moved to a local restaurant for a most enjoyable lunch followed by the trip to Newgrange a place we had wished to visit for many years but never got around to it. We had a most enjoyable night at the banquet and finished up obtaining two upper stand tickets for the hurling final on the following day between Kilkenny and Offaly. It was a one-sided match won by Kilkenny. However the minor curtain raiser made my day by Galway minors defeating Cork.

After walking back to the hotel we took a taxi to Aidan and Maura's reception to complete a most enjoyable weekend and celebration. It was encouraging to see so many of us still around despite the inevitable loss of twenty-four over forty-eight years.

When the reunion ended we decided that those of us who would survive for another two years would return to our alma mater in Belfield for the official Golden Jubilee in September 2002. This took place on 20th September that year as planned.

My original intention was to finish the story of my life, From Slyne Head to Malin Head, A Rural GP Remembers, at the end of our millennium reunion but changing circumstances have convinced me that I should add an epilogue.

Epilogue

Around 1995 – 96 our family and myself noticed slight changes in Eileen's personality. She became more forgetful and repeated questions more frequently than normal but this was not obvious to people outside the family.

While she was still driving her car and playing golf, medical investigation concluded that she was showing very early signs of Alzheimer's disease.

Aricept, the first drug claimed to slow down the progress of the disease in the early stages, was tried and it did appear to have a marginal slowing down effect on the progress of the symptoms for about two years.

This was around the time that I was involved with the presidency of the ICGP and she was delighted to travel with me north, south, east and west attending dinners and various other functions.

She appeared to enjoy every minute of it and kept up talk and banter at top tables of numerous dinners where invited presidents and spouses were invariably seated. We continued our usual routines of swimming up to five days per week in the pool also walking and going to any musicals or concerts in the old Rialto in Derry.

As time went on deterioration became more obvious and accelerated more rapidly. She had difficulty in locating different shops and in recognising people until eventually she had to be close to me at all times.

By December 2000 she could not find the changing room in the pool and from then went downhill until Saturday the 7th July 2001. That day we had a meal out which was almost a daily routine and at that stage, in mid-summer, she was going to bed between seven and eight pm. Around 3 am on Sunday 8th July I got a severe heart attack. Fortunately I was able to call the Moville Health Centre to get a GP who happened to be my former colleague and friend Dr Don McGinley. He ordered the ambulance and came to my assistance very rapidly and the ambulance arrived a very short time later. At this stage Eileen was very confused and had no idea of what was going on. After having the usual emergency treatment I was wheeled into the ambulance while Eileen sat in the front with the driver for the speedy eighteen mile journey to the coronary care in Atlnagelvin Hospital in Derry. We were certainly very fortunate to have two sons and their wives practising GPs in the Derry area so the two sons were at the hospital when we arrived.

I made a satisfactory recovery and did not require a by-pass but had an angioplast. Eileen deteriorated and required permanent care in a home.

While all this was a very traumatic experience and life will never be the same again it could have been much worse. Seeing Eileen in her present state is stressful but I am grateful that we had a reasonably long life together and we had the great blessing to see our family grow up to marry and have successful lives and have given us grandchildren.

My real loss is the companionship, which we enjoyed so much since our retirement the swimming in the pool, the gardening, walking on the local beaches and the big loss of the musical shows in Derry. Our eleven years of blissful retirement were certainly a long way better than none.